Extreme Rapid weig

for wor

Regain the control of your body. You'll Find: Powerful
Gastric band hypnosis, affirmations, guided meditations, mini habits, intermittent fasting for woman 50

D.R. Thompson

Table of Contents

Introduction

The Journal of Health Economics provides quite $ 200 billion annually within us for medical obesity research costs. Consistent with SAD (Standard American Diet), processed foods and beverages high in fat, sodium, and sugar spread to other countries, increasing heart condition, diabetes, and other life-threatening problems. The food industry has been treating overweight people for many years - most of the people have tried various diets and other programs that either fail or work temporarily and have made them even more discouraged.

You will find plenty of help books that offer you diet plans, but they're useless. If you question this, when trying to satisfy the diet's requirements, including allowing all of the ingredients, you'll reduce with only the trouble required to follow the diet. But here is that the most crucial statistic that anyone who wants to reduce should know. Most of the people who reduce successfully continue a diet and gain even more weight within the first year! These statistics include people that have participated within the Biggest Loser or whose stomachs are stapled. This way is often the foremost suppressed statistic within the food industry: only 3 in 100 people that reach their goal manage to take care of this weight loss beyond the first year.

A post-mortem with the remainder of the 97 people that struggled to stay their burden showed that they were much hungry after trying their regular diet again than they were before the load loss program. They need been busy eating since the top of their diet, and a few are crazy about food.

From the attitude of human evolution, eating is that the phenomenon of the last second. Historically telling, the 1920s was a mere failure to market less eating, but as a society, the cycle of dietary habits that triggered famine brain mechanisms began until the late 1960s.

A weight-loss diet, by definition, requires a discount in food intake below what the body must maintain its current form. There's no real food shortage, but all the built-in mechanisms that ensure our survival record fat loss. This reduction triggers a neural circuit that uses a military of hormones that cause the order of overeating. This mechanism is just called the famine brain.

Overeating works because of the brain's primary reward system for dieting. Unfortunately, researchers have found that weight loss of all types uses our neurochemical weapons. If you've got an excessive amount of fat, your body won't know. It only "knows" if you risk losing fat. During a bold plan to regain homeostasis, our system lowers the hormone levels that signal satiety (leptin and insulin) and pumps the fasting hormone 'ghrelin' into the bloodstream. This hormone leads to heightened looking for food resulting in extra calorie intake and eventually more weight gain.

Scientists aren't yet conscious of how the brain and physical starvation system interact to support or override one another. What we all know is that a lot of regular diets cause a mind hooked into food. Therefore, the basis of the matter lies within the brain, where this cycle continues.

The way we will save us from this cycle is to optimize brain activity. This optimization and control are what you'll learn during this book.

Thankfully, we will change our brain patterns to behave differently. During this book, we'll study self-hypnosis, cognitive behavioral therapy, sleep learning system, and meditation to regulate our brain and overcome food cravings. To quickly put, we'll optimize brain activity.

Chapter 1

Introduction to Gastric Band Hypnosis

The gastric band is an adjustable silicone device utilized in bariatric surgery. The group is placed around the upper part of the stomach to make a pouch above the machine. This limits the quantity of food stored in the stomach, making it challenging to consume in large quantities. Stomach banding aims to limit the quantity of food an individual can eat to feel full after eating little or no food to encourage weight loss. For many people undergoing this operation, this is often the last option after trying other weight loss methods. Like all surgery, there are risks in installing a gastric band.

Gastric Band Hypnosis

Gastric hypnosis can help people reduce the danger of surgery. Many hypnotherapists use a two-pronged approach. First, they specialize in determining the basis of explanation for your emotional diet. With hypnosis, the therapist can encourage you to recollect long-forgotten experiences with food, affecting you subconsciously. By hypnotizing stomach bands, it's going to help resolve and identify any unhealthy thinking patterns surrounding food. Next, the hypnotherapy; the therapist will perform virtual gastric band therapy. This procedure is meant to suggest at a subconscious level that you have completed surgery to insert a gastric band. The aim is to make your body answer this recommendation and make it feel faster as if you had performed a true surgery.

Mini Gastric-band

This process is suitable for patrons who got to reduce the load of 30 pounds (15Kgs). It's going to be that you simply have lost weight but have reached a balanced state. This therapy is ideal for those that wish to change bad eating habits. Maybe you're a "yoyo weight loss" and wish to interrupt the cycle. This treatment isn't suitable for those that got to reduce. The Mini Stomach Band gives you a sense of "satisfaction" and may prevent many of us from overeating. We can also get to address cravings. Every client will respond differently and consistent with their habits, but this treatment should cause you to feel satisfied with a small meal and not crave more.

There are two stages to the treatment:

• Free consultation for half-hour

• Therapeutic session and mini-band "implantation." (Gastric contraction) (Up to three hours a day)

After treatment, it'll provide you with:

Email backup

• 2 x 15 minutes' phone backup

• If necessary, you'll enjoy a 50% discount to optimize your treatment.

• Whole stomach band

The Quanwei Band is meant for those that have lost quite two stones (13 kg). It aims to eliminate some bad eating behaviors, such as:

• No meals, especially breakfast or lunch

• Overeating while eating, controlling diet

• Must clean dishes (and other dishes)

• Snacks, picking, and grazing "munches."

• Craving for food - sugar, chocolate, cakes, biscuits, sausage rolls, etc.

• Junk food and takeaway

• Fast food

The treatment is split into three stages:

• Free consultation (30 minutes)

• Treatment time (up to 4 hours a day) (including stomach contractions)

- One follow-up adjustment After treatment, it'll provide you with:
- Email backup
- 2 x 15 minutes' phone backup
- If necessary, you'll make longer changes to enjoy a 50% discount to perfect your medicine.

How It Works

A hypnotherapist using relaxation techniques will put you into a hypnotic state. And in this relaxed environment, your subconscious is more likely to accept suggestions.

By now, the hypnotherapist will make recommendations to your subconscious. When performing hypnosis treatment for stomach bands, this means that you have installed an environmental group. Your mind is powerful, so if your subconscious accepts these suggestions, your behavior will change accordingly. Usually, alongside the "fitting" of the virtual stomach band, recommendations about confidence and action will help you plan lifestyle changes. Several therapists will also teach self- hypnosis techniques so that you'll strengthen your work after the meeting.

It's also often recommended to self-educate nutrition and exercise to market physical health and well-being.

Your first meeting with a hypnotherapist could also be a preliminary consultation, where you discuss what you would like from hypnosis. This is often a chance to debate any previous weight loss attempts, your eating habits, any health issues, and your general attitude towards food.

This information will make the therapist know more clearly what's helpful and whether the other sorts of treatment should be considered.

The tactic itself is meant to mimic gastric band surgery to help your subconscious believe that it indeed happened. To make the experience more real, many hypnotists will combine the sound and smell of the OR. Your therapist will first put you into a state of deep relaxation, also referred to as hypnosis, you'll know what happened, and you'll always be on top of things.

Once you're hypnotized, the therapist will discuss the procedure with you. They're going to gradually introduce things in the operation, starting with anesthesia, making the primary incision, fixing the Band-Aid itself, then suture the incision. The sound and smell of the OR will enhance the experience and persuade your subconscious of what's happening to you. As mentioned earlier, other suggestions are often added in the procedure to extend self-confidence. After the method is completed, your hypnosis therapist may teach you some self-hypnosis skills to help you retain your pace reception. Some hypnotherapists will ask you to return for follow-up appointments to watch the virtual band's success and make any adjustments. This happens when people also install physical tapes. For a few people, continuing hypnotherapy as a part of a long-term weight management plan may help. And this enables the hypnotherapist to figure with you to unravel potential problems surrounding food and self-esteem.

Stomach band hypnosis should make part of a weight management program that focuses on nutrition and exercise habits. For those that seek to reduce, it's usually the habit of adjusting the body and mind that's generally the foremost successful.

How Will I Feel?

The overall goal of gastric hypnosis is to market a healthy relationship with food. When your subconscious thinks you've worn a stomach band, it'll feel that your stomach is smaller. In turn, this causes your brain to send a message that you simply are full after eating less food. For those that are overeating, it isn't easy to acknowledge once you are full. Sometimes, we eat purely for tasting (or comfort) and ignore whether we are hungry.

Learning to acknowledge the physiological sensations of hunger and satiety helps develop healthy eating habits. Unlike gastric band surgery, virtual stomach bands don't have any physical side effects.

For some people, real medicine may cause nausea, vomiting, and acid reflux. Because stomach hypnosis isn't a physical process, it doesn't cause this symptom. This process should be a pleasing and relaxing experience, and most of the people will feel calm after hypnosis.

Does It Work for Me?

For those that try hypnosis for the primary time, a standard question is: Does it work for me? Unfortunately, this is often not an easy "yes" or "no" situation; it mostly depends on you. Hypnosis can help people with various problems, but it's especially useful in changing habits. Therefore, it can successfully help people develop healthy eating habits and reduce weight. However, like all other weight loss systems, this may require your full investment.

If you think about this process and your therapist, you're more likely to request what you would like from stomach band hypnosis therapy. It's essential to be comfortable and trust your hypnotherapist. This is why it's recommended that you spend a while researching hypnotherapy therapists in the area to find out more about them, how they work, and also the qualifications needed. You should plan to meet them before the operation to make sure you're comfortable with them. If you're committed to changing your lifestyle, please believe this procedure and your hypnotherapist. Stomach band hypnosis should serve you.

What Is Involved in Hypnosis Treatment of Gastric Band?

Like any other hypnosis program, stomach band hypnosis starts with a deep relaxation protocol designed to make your body and mind as relaxed as possible. Once you're relaxed, the hypnotist will use a piece of strong advice- based script to make your subconscious pretend that you are simply undergoing gastric bypass surgery. The essential concept here is that the subconscious doesn't understand the difference between reality and imagination. If you'll convince the subconscious to do something, then the subconscious will bring success.

To persuade your subconscious, the hypnotist may even use smells and sounds associated with the hospital environment. This may be combined with strong post-hypnosis recommendations so that your stomach can only eat a little amount of food from now on.

What Does Stomach Band Hypnosis Involve?

Stomach band hypnosis may be a course-based therapy; you'd not expect to be "cured" in one course. We expect 4-5 meetings to figure the best in a period. Confine your mind that most behavioral patterns, including overeating and poor eating, is got to "go" from our system. Stomach Band Hypnosis works together with your subconscious to retrain potential behavioral habits. You should consider that although we take 4-5 sessions on average, everyone is different, and therefore the required treatment depth will vary.

Once your hypnotist therapist evaluates your problems and wishes that you comply with continued treatment, an entire history record will be created for your files. Stomach band hypnosis therapy also requires auxiliary activities, and you'll hope that it'll provide MP3 or CD to reinforce your subconscious cues.

Do You Want to Lose Weight?

Thousands of individuals desire what you are doing now. Christmas has passed, the celebrations have brought some additional burdens, and therefore the drinking festival seems to continue. But at heart, you recognize that you simply aren't very satisfied with what happened, and you would like to vary it. So far, the diet might not assist you, but you're willing to undertake something which will offer you a particular advantage to regulate your food cravings. If you're getting to try hypnotherapy, why not download my free e-book, explaining why dieting alone doesn't provide the results you usually wanted. Allow us to discuss the staged hypnosis and gastric hypnosis.

Stage performances use hypnosis as a way of entertaining the audience. The people on stage are usually volunteers, they know what they're doing, or they're curious, and they want to have fun. The recommendation they followed only targeted the performance's background and was deleted in hypnosis. One of the differences between stage hypnosis and therapeutic hypnosis is suggested after using hypnosis. Usually, a sound stage hypnotist will provide volunteers with hypnosis advice for energy, health, and honest sleep before awakening them. After hypnosis, the recommendation provided is deeper, and the consciousness involved is smaller. In therapeutic hypnosis, it is advised to use anesthesia at an appropriate depth so that you'll make the changes you would like because they're natural.

You Didn't Know About Gastric Band

My first impression is that I should tell you that gastric hypnosis isn't for everybody. I mean, it's not for everybody. The foremost successful patients are those that want to vary their weight, eating habits, and dietary relationships. Those trying to find crutches, or simply reaching out so that they do not need to use themselves, are unlikely to achieve by the end of the day. Hypnosis advice is best for those with the proper mindset. Although this doesn't mean that stomach band hypnosis won't work for you, each situation depends on its advantages and drawbacks.

To undertake or point out fairness throughout the method, be happy to see out some video recommendations and feedback from colleagues in Australia. Below I will mention five belongings you do not know about hypnotism, which you ought to understand. You do not need to have a stomach band before having the understanding.

This may seem obvious, but I received calls from some people that confuse stomach band hypnosis therapy with the particular medical procedures provided by a personal person or the NHS.

Hypnosis bands are the foremost common practice of stomach hypnosis and don't involve surgery. Hypnosis therapy may be a non-invasive sort of weight loss hypnosis therapy, which achieves the specified effect through suggestive and cognitive behavioral therapy. If you've got any of the above fears, you do not need to attend the hospital, see the doctor, or nurse.

Does It Work for Me?

Gastric hypnosis depends on you. You would like to be committed to reducing the load of the top and heart. This solution isn't suitable for those seeking "other things to regulate." You're the key to your success! Candidates must be prepared to change their eating habits and overall lifestyle habits. If quite one person in your family is suitable for this treatment, please consider whether the person isn't prepared to change their practices. If you regularly trigger and prompt to eat tons of inappropriate food, this might have an immediate impact on your results. If you're serious about losing weight, then it'll work for you.

Can Stomach Band Hypnosis Guarantee Me to Lose Weight?

Due to various factors that will affect surgery or practice, any clinic doesn't provide any specific guarantees for the results. One thing we will confirm is that gastric band hypnosis doesn't cause any therapeutic side effects. You want to remember that in any hypnosis, quitting smoking, fear of height, or spiders, the result depends on the individual; that's you! If you're not 100% interested, hypnotherapy won't work.

You want to understand that the mind may be a very complex and powerful organ, and by performing stomach band hypnosis therapy, you'll get the required tools to arm yourself to change your old eating habits. The treatment is meant to improve your mindset and lifestyle to change your relationship with food and reduce.

What Should I Expect from The Treatment?

Process?

The stomach band hypnosis treatment includes an evaluation period and a treatment period of several hours. We usually support this function through CD or MP3 recording to further improve the treatment level. An honest therapist will fully record your diet and medical record before any treatment. In the first treatment, you'll be introduced to hypnosis, which is an enhanced learning state, and you'll also feel extremely relaxed and calm. In the next lesson, you'll be introduced to the hypnotherapeutics of the gastric band, and your hypnotherapist will work with you to "adapt" to the virtual gastric band to urge the foremost out of it. Future courses will introduce your relationship with food and eating habits.

Chapter 2

Benefits

Gastric banding is taken into account the safest bariatric surgery. This is often a comparatively simple, low-risk, minimally invasive procedure with few complications. Compared with other gastric surgery, gastric band surgery usually shortens the hospital stay (only one night). The recovery time is quicker (about a week). The scars are smaller, and therefore, the pain is a smaller amount. Unlike gastric bypass surgery and sleeve gastrectomy, gastric banding doesn't permanently change your body, such as removing a part of your stomach or rerouting and sewing your body. It's completely reversible and may be deleted as required. Fastening the stomach band won't interfere with the digestion and absorption of food. Vitamin deficiency and dumping syndrome, which are usually related to gastric bypass surgery, are unlikely to occur through the gastric band, so you do not need to take nutritional supplements a day. You'll easily and quickly adjust to the strap in your surgeon's clinic or hospital to assist you in mastering the progress of weight loss. The gastric band features a more gradual weight loss effect than other gastric surgery. Losing weight can make it easier for you to maneuver around, perform daily activities, and participate in new activities that help improve your overall health.

Losing weight with a gastric band can improve comorbidities related to obesity, including type 2 diabetes, high cholesterol, apnea, and high vital sign. After weight loss through gastric banding surgery, you'll feel that your psychological state has improved, self-esteem and physical self-esteem have increased, depression symptoms are reduced, and quality of life has improved.

The gastric band will make a little bag ahead of the stomach, trapped when the food is ingested. The advantage of this is that it can often reduce the capacity of solid food, and other people will eat faster. The food in the sachet digests more slowly, so an individual's "fullness" can last long after a meal. Studies have shown that this method can reduce a mean of 23 kg of weight at two years and a mean of 43 kg of weight at five years. And most patients who attempt to reduce without this surgery won't lose any weight for an extended time. Laparoscopic ligation is taken into account as the safest of all weight loss procedures.

In most cases, patients will only be hospitalized for twenty-four hours. After the operation, many obesity-related diseases improved. Studies conducted two years after laparoscopic ligation surgery has shown that the effect of laparoscopic surgery has improved:

- Blood pressure
- Cholesterol
- Asthma

- Diabetes
- Gastroesophageal reflux
- Heart failure
- Sleep apnea
- Depression
- Infertility
- Blood clot.

Risks

Inserting a gastric band may be a surgery, and although there are few potential risks, there are also some side effects of stomach bands worth nothing. The most complications which will occur after stomach weight loss surgery include infection, blood clots in the legs (deep vein thrombosis) or lungs (pulmonary embolism), and internal bleeding. Usually, every tenth person will need further surgery in the future, and this might be for a spread of reasons. Your wound, port, or wristband may be infected and should get to be repositioned, replaced, or removed. Sometimes, your wristband may enter or undergo the stomach wall very slowly to invalidate it, so it must be removed and replaced.

Over time, the band may slip, and therefore the stomach pouch will become more abundant. Your gastric band must be fixed in the correct position. The components of the gastric band may separate tanks to damage and cause leakage. Damaged parts will get to get replaced. Some stomach bands can develop food intolerance, resulting in symptoms like nausea, vomiting, and esophageal reflux (GER). In most cases, avoiding foods because of reactions will help, but if you've got persistent symptoms associated with many various foods, it's going to be necessary to get rid of the wristband. People that reduce have a high risk of gallstone formation regardless of which sort of stomach weight loss surgery they use.

Laparoscopic gastric ring ligation surgery is more complicated than other sorts of surgery. However, most surgeons performing this operation are experienced. The surgeon performing this procedure should discuss the complications with you before the service. The general incidence of complications is additionally very low. The danger of death from this operation is shallow, but 0.5%. Like any sort of surgery, there's little risk of infection, wound problems, blood clots, or lung problems. There are measures to scale back these complications that your doctor may prescribe. There's a risk of the belt slipping or the bag inflating. These problems may require further surgery in approximately 25% of cases. In about 2% of the population, rubber bands may erode the stomach wall. After the operation, some patients will experience vomiting associated with diet. This condition doesn't happen to all patients and may be reduced by eating a little amount. This process has not always been successful. A couple of patients won't reduce through this operation. However, in patients with rapid weight loss, there's a risk of developing gallbladder inflammation, which can require gallbladder removal.

Using Gastric Band for Weight Loss

No Strict Juice or Powder Detox

It sounds strange because wherever you go and stand, a detox juice cure is being advertised, but it doesn't add up to be consistent with nutritionists and an expert's prescriptions. Consistent with this, an excessively strict detox regimen in which nothing is consumed for an extended period aside from juices or maybe mixed powder drinks also can cause devastating damage to the body and is therefore rather unhealthy than healthy. Everything that ought to cause you to happier, healthier, leaner, and more energetic in seven days should be questioned. You save your wallet if you retain your hands off such expensive treatments.

No Bans

Anyone who has already been on a diet knows that when certain foods are banned, you would like to eat them even more! If you then have an evil conscience, you're more inclined to eat all the chocolate directly because after taking a bit of the "forbidden fruit," it doesn't matter anymore. Therefore, a complete ban on less healthy foods is pointless and can sooner or later cause a relapse. Instead, enjoy here and there and still not lose sight of the goal.

Step by Step

Those who want to reduce their diet to change their eating habit at some point sometimes and suddenly have to empty unhealthy diet. That's what often makes many fail! Therefore, experts advise you to gradually change your eating habits step by step, a primary meal, then secondary, and so on. It's best to think beforehand about which meal change has a major significant effect on the specified goal.

Always Slow

Exercise is simply as important as nutrition to remain healthy, to become healthy, or to reduce. Those who decide to attend sports five times every week and provide full power will quickly reach their limits. Those who haven't done games before or want to start again after an extended time should slowly take it and increase it step by step. Attend fitness twice every week, then three times after four weeks then on. And perhaps not just choose the facility cycling course, but swing on the treadmill.

Eat just for Special Occasions

If you cook in the house, you've got to switch how healthy or unhealthy the plate is. So, if you would like to drop weight, you ought to prepare yourself tons. Eating out is somewhat tricky because you never know which products are used and, above all, which unnecessary, unhealthy additives are included. Eating at a restaurant should be an exception and reserved for special occasions - but this will be the weekend. Those that have a stressful lifestyle tend to postpone the workout again instead of roll in the hay. It pays to make a to-do list that gives a detailed overview of the daily workload and available time for a training session. Planning also helps to do what you've got done ultimately.

Healthy Snacks

During the day, one often tends to snack on something here and there. Often you're not starving in the least, but boredom, then a chocolate candy quickly lands in the mouth, and therefore the Haribo bag is open. Listen carefully to yourself. Are you hungry and can't stand it? Or are you only bored because you've got three hours to figure and zip to do? If there's absolutely no snack, confirm to eat the proper thing in between. A couple of tomatoes, a sugar-free cookie, or an apple work wonders.

Water in Its Place of sentimental Drinks

Probably the simplest method to save lots of calories is to reduce soft drinks and drink water. That's not only good for the scales but also for the insulin level, which is no longer pushed continuously up and causes seizures after the rapid decline. Those that are "addicted" to sweetened drinks (including sugar in coffee!) should swap one for the opposite step by step. It doesn't need to be three coke, just maybe one.

Strength Training

No question, regardless of what sport, it's better than no game. It's not fair that cardio training, which has preached forever, always reaps all the laurels because strength training ensures muscle build- up, stimulating metabolism, and burning more calories. So rather than stand up on the treadmill for 3 hours, you better hold dumbbells in your hand and do strength training.

Stairs rather than An Elevator

You often need to motivate yourself to travel to the gym. Small exercises are so obvious! Whether reception or in the office, just use the steps rather than the elevator. Find like-minded people and role models, those that fight alone often surrender more quickly because nobody sees it! So, it's best to look for like-minded people with whom you would like to reduce, cook, and motivate yourself. But a task model also can help! Why not just speak to an excellent, well-trained woman in the gym and ask if she will support you?

Correct Portion Sizes

Do you know what you ate today? And that is precisely the matter. Often you simply overeat without even knowing it; otherwise, you underestimate the portion sizes. Weighing and keeping a diary helps immensely to urge a summary of what you eat throughout the day.

Green Vegetables

You should involve green vegetables in your food a minimum of 3 times each day. It contains many essential nutrients and is additionally filling. Green vegetables are too high for healthy green smoothies!

Legumes

If you've got a rare kilo too abundant on your hips, you're guaranteed not to eat enough fruit, vegetables, and legumes. The latter is incredibly healthy! They contain tons of fiber, fill you up, and supply the body with valuable nutrients. Refraining from meat also has an economically beneficial effect.

Drink rather than eating

Everyone knows this sense of being close to starving. Our brain often plays a trick on us in sugar craze. Also, you usually confuse hunger with thirst if you drink insufficient water! So, if you think that you're hungry, you ought to first drink a glass of water. If that does not help and therefore, the last meal is five hours or more to go, you should safely eat something.

Smaller Plates

Psychology features a firm grip on us. The plate should be full; otherwise, we'll not be complete. Nobody said how big the plate should be. So, if you would like to outsmart yourself, you should always put your portions on a little plate. It's sort of a lot, but it's less!

No Temptations

Honestly: If you've got nutriment and sweets in the house, you'll eat them at some point! The temptation is particularly significant once you feel hungry and need to devour something. However, if you initially need to leave the house for sinful food, you're more inclined to eat what's in sight - ideally healthy food. You simply need to resist temptation in the supermarket!

Strength rather than weight

If you set your goals on gaining strength instead of weight loss, you'll hold out longer! The Plank Challenge is right for this. Just start with a plank today and do another day. You'll notice physical changes quickly, if not on the scales.

Eat More Fat

That may sound insane for several, but fat isn't only a flavor carrier; it also keeps you full for an extended time and is healthy - as long as they're the right fats. Often make an avocado in the smoothie, sprinkle nuts over the salad, or drink a bulletproof coffee, and therefore the change in diet is suddenly not that difficult anymore.

Healthy Snacks for the Movie Evening

Do not tempt yourself - with the good snacks, you'll roll in the hay at the film evening together with your best friends or partner. Rather than chips, chocolate, and gummy bears, peppers, cucumber, and curd can sweeten the evening. If you fancy chocolate, you'll treat yourself to a touch of bittersweet chocolate with a minimum of 80 percent.

Do Not believe, Greens!

It sounds illogical but true; studies show that if you think that you're eating "light" food, you'll not feel full. And it isn't just psychology; your thoughts about eating can cause you to compute more ghrelin hormone, which prevents your feeling of fullness. Therefore, rather than brooding about greens in your salad, better believe it's more high-calorie part: cheese, avocado, nuts. It also helps to settle on healthy foods but bring pleasure, like a delicious broth or lemon- garlic shrimp with vegetables.

Include Your Partner in the Process

Losing weight will be quite tricky if your partner eats cakes and desserts, so include them in the process. Let him (or her) know that you simply need his support, and if you regularly attend restaurants or buy takeaway food, then attempt to do research and choose healthier options: maybe not buying (or halving) dessert, spend time for a joint workout. If you attract your partner (and are firm about your own intention to lose weight), losing weight will be much easier.

Do not dine in Front of the TV.

Firstly, studies have repeatedly shown that there's a correlation between obesity and hanging call in front of the TV - this is often why the expression appeared: "Idler and celery won't help." Studies have shown that folks who eat while watching TV consume a mean of 280 more calories. Every additional 2 hours of watching TV per day adds 23% to the likelihood of obesity.

And not only that: if you watch TV, then you are doing no practice and not sleeping at this point. So, eat only at the table, do small workouts in the advertising, and replace the TV hour with the hour of drills - if you follow these rules a day, you'll be closer and closer to your goal.

Eat More Fiber

Adequate fiber in your diet is important for weight loss. That's one of the critical tools for effective weight loss. Why? Due to it, you feel full-fiber absorbs water and expands in your stomach, which, in turn, contributes to the assembly of leptin, a hormone that provides a sense of satiety. Find several sources of fiber that you love and eat daily. Try broccoli, flaxseeds, and apples!

Train Hard

Studies have shown that short but high-intensity workouts burn more calories than long ones with moderate intensity. In other words, walking on a treadmill isn't the simplest way to lose weight. A quarter-hour of high-intensity exercise is far more useful than 1 hour of slow cardio. One of our favorite ways is to leap rope; at Harvard school of medicine, an individual weighing 57 kilograms will burn 300 kcal in half-hour. Remember that you got to increase the intensity of your workouts slowly and gradually. It'll be even better if you consult your doctor before making changes to your exercise or diet.

Combine Workout and Diet

Only training won't provide a good result; Choosing between two healthy diets is far more important (although you want to combine both parts with being genuinely healthy). Because the saying goes, you can't "over-train" (correct with training) a bad diet. So, eat healthy foods and find an exercise that you simply like. Then you'll be on your way to your ideal healthy weight.

Ignore Spontaneous Purchases

Everything in the malls is meant for you to spare your money. All the windows pack to the brim with chocolates, soda, and other all types of saboteurs of your weight loss. Marketers know that this momentary weakness is for people. Studies have shown that such spontaneous purchases amount to over 14,000 calories consumed per woman per year! Not only do these sudden purchases hit your wallet, but they also contribute to your fullness!

The good news is that after you learn this little trick, it'll be much easier to resist it. Just think: "That is trying to require my money and make me fat!". Then you only close your eyes and proudly travel by. Don't forget to double-check yourself because further research shows that the amount of such sudden purchases will decrease by 32% if you only check your grocery cart.

Do Not concentrate on Strict Diets and Magic Pills.

Losing and maintaining weight (this is a crucial part) requires a lifestyle change, but you ought to not change everything at once: just by making small healthy steps a day, you'll meet up with and closer to your goal. The most thing to know is that you simply must make long-term changes. Strict diets and diet pills work just for a brief distance (but can have adverse consequences for your health).

Often people, in the end, only return to their original weight, then you've got to start everywhere again once you want to reduce again! Let your health become a habit. Making small healthy decisions a day, you'll begin to enjoy the method, and it'll be much easier to realize success.

Disable Cravings for Food

All desires begin with something: it is often a sort of sweet glaze or a delicious chicken flavor. On an emotional level, a pie will offer you a way of comfort just because memories of the house are related to it. Or, for instance, you'll associate the top of the workweek with Chinese food. So, ultimately, you'll crave this particular food when you actually need the sensation that's related to it. For instance, you would like pie once you had a bad day. You do not need food; rather, you need emotions.

Next time you would like, try another way: believe the emotion you're trying to seek out in food. And check out to seek out differently to that, on which there's no food. If you can't immediately satisfy this emotion completely, attempt to make it in small steps, if possible.

Clean Your Surroundings

If you're determined to reduce, you would like to vary the sources where you get ideas for cooking. Hide cookbooks, find several books with healthy dishes, put them on your cocktail table, obviate a substantial amount of frozen dessert, and obviate a large amount of frozen diet spread on muffins. Watch healthy eating programs and skip unnecessary food commercials. Ignore marketing; specialize in your weight loss. Avoid treats at work and notify your colleagues that you simply are losing weight and eating healthy (but remember that everything depends on you). In other words, shop around and announce: "There may be a new sheriff in this city!" Hire a private trainer.

Sometimes it's easier to motivate yourself if someone kicks you. Not only for that. You'll also find out how to do the exercises correctly and warm-up and funky down so that there are no injuries. A private trainer is often an upscale pleasure, but it might be nice to urge a specific educational program from an expert—Cook less food at a time.

When you cook, you want to eat. It's sometimes better to chop back on a number of the planned dishes, which can bring you even closer to the goal.

Find Other Sources of Emotion

Have you heard about the comfort of food? Emotional eaters often address food to satisfy their passionate thirst. Usually, these are high-calorie, sweet, fatty foods in other words. That's what you would like to avoid in other to lose excess weight. Truthfully, once you address food to deal with stress or boredom, it'll not help you eliminate negative feelings. Things often worsen.

The solution is often to seek out an explanation for your emotional eating and make positive changes in this area. It might be your job or relationship, maybe something else. Until then, make an inventory of activities not associated with food. What might be a step towards satisfying your emotional needs: running, watching comedy shows, talking with friends, reading anything. If you discover something which will move you to a healthy state, you'll get another good push towards your goal. Use online support.

There are many great communities on the web that help people that want to reduce. So, no matter your goals (expressed in specific kilograms of desired weight loss), register in communities, and participate in their lives. Remember that in the end, it all depends on you, and you'll roll in the hay.

Recount

Most people underestimate the number of calories they consume and overestimate the number of calories they burn. That's why keeping a food journal is often your ally for losing weight. If something enters your stomach, write it down. Measure everything at the very starting to get an accurate picture of how healthy the portions look, or use recipes that you recognize precisely the amount of calories per serving. What happens once you start doing this? You'll begin to develop an awareness of the percentage of calories you consume. Pay special attention to high-calorie foods, and you'll eat a spread of sauces, salad dressings, fruits, etc.

Another mistake could also be to overestimate the number of calories you burn in this exercise. For instance, if you exercise for half an hour on a treadmill, then burn about 300 calories, you'll head home and think: "I am well trained; I can click and eat a few of cookies." Yes, you'll eat some cookies late, thereby destroying the full effect of the workout. So, spend time and concentrate on what percentage of calories you consume and how much you burn in training. Don't forget to record it!

Find Convenient Sources of Protein

We already told you ways protein helps you reduce, but most protein sources are very uncomfortable. Therefore, confirm that you simply always have a snack available containing an excessive amount of protein, if possible—some good choices like boiled eggs, protein powder, nuts, or jerky. Keeping your protein high also will make sure that you lose fat, not muscle.

Get used to Eating Low Glucose.

Studies have shown that diets with reduced glucose intake have a big effect on weight loss (especially for women). In one study, reduced glucose intake doubled the loss of fat compared to a gaggle of subjects who ate high glucose. So, try soup, snack on bananas, or try the other low-glucose meal.

Chew More Thoroughly

Studies have shown that folks with healthy weight chew on average 15 times, while overweight people, on average, 12 times; therefore, attempt to eat more thoroughly. That slows down your meals and activates many digestive processes, and allows you to feel the natural food taste, which means that you simply are less likely to urge extra calories from seasonings.

Eat More Protein

Eat high-quality protein with every meal. Studies have shown that protein helps maintain muscle mass and reduces body fat while you're losing weight. Also, the protein contains an excessive amount of YY Peptide (PYY), which suppresses appetite. But confirm that this is often a part of a diet because more than protein gives a high load on the kidneys (and not only). So, don't ditch vegetables!

Do not Overeat fruit.

Everyone loves fruit. An excellent healthy alternative to sweets is the fruit, but moderation is required. Nuts are filled with various natural sugars. For instance, grapes are made entirely of sugar. There's some evidence that sweet fruits cause you to feel hungry.

So, moderate the consumption of fruits - don't overeat them. Try low- sugar fruits and replace some fruits with vegetables in your diet. Try a snack of fresh peas, slices of cucumber, celery, or whatever you would like. Attempt to get the maximum amount as possible from fruits, use them as an authoritative source of energy.

Lift Weights

If you build muscle, then your rate will increase. This means that you simply will burn more calories even once you aren't exercising. You'll not only improve your body shape and be more toned but also will burn fats, a bit like that. If you're a lady, then you shouldn't worry that you simply will grow huge muscles - this is often a myth (women don't have natural testosterone). Yes, some useful tips for losing weight. Not so obvious or intuitive: studies have found that once you lift 85% of your maximum load, then in 8 repetitions, you'll burn eight times more calories than once you lift less weight with an excessive number of repetitions. In other words, lift weights (but not too heavy).

Note that strength exercises aren't necessarily related to lifting some quite large barbells. For instance, lunges on one leg are

recommended on this page. Put aside your cutlery after each bite. Most folks eat in no time, right? The matter is that it should take about 20 minutes after starting a meal before the instant your brain informs you that you are full. In other words, once you eat too fast, the brain doesn't have enough time to inform you: "Hey, wait, the tank is already full." once you erode a slower pace, you give your brain time to send signals, which will assist you not to overeat.

Stay Away From "Porn" with Food

Everyone likes to check out pictures with tasty, eye-catching, sweet, and mouth-watering food, but they understand that they ought not to eat it. But neuroscientists have found that dalliance viewing of such images provokes your emotional and physical hunger. True! Even worse, they found that folks with a predisposition to overweight are even more sensitive to the consequences of viewing images with food. Research has also found that viewing food images increases your ghrelin (a hormone that creates the feeling when hungry). Furthermore, studies have shown that folks with this habit are more susceptible to overeating than those that check out real food ahead of them! So, stand back from this food porn or try healthier options: images of a healthy diet or exercise.

Do not Eat While Standing

Studies have shown that folks tend to eat faster once they roll in the hay while standing, i.e., outside the board. When viewed at a psychological level, it's much easier to underestimate such mini-snacks compared to meals at the table. As a result, we move far away from our food intake schedule and that we consume more tons of calories - this is often bad for losing weight. It's good that you eat once you are hungry so as to maintain a perfect healthy weight. In the meantime, you want to reorganize yourself to a healthier diet. Until you reach the goal, if you discover yourself eating while standing, you'll presumably not eat now (if this is often not a healthy snack). So, save this meal for your planned meal.

Do It Slowly

As the saying goes: "If you've got not hung out on this, then don't await the result." Studies have repeatedly shown that the foremost successful approach to reducing and maintaining weight may be a slow and measured approach. If you strive to lose a kilogram per week, you'll only burn fat, but not muscle. Don't attend grocery stores when you are hungry.

You must understand why. Once you go out hungry, you would like to place everything in your basket—especially sweet and salty things. There's a reason for this: studies have shown that the brain signals that you simply choose high-calorie foods once you are hungry. It'll be delicious, of course, but not for your weight loss. So, to remain on target, following a healthy lifestyle, have a snack before getting to the shop, or eat healthy food before shopping.

Use vegetable oil

You may already have the proper skill of the Mediterranean diet because it has a high amount of protein, abundant vegetables, and healthy fats. It seems that vegetable oil also features a significant role in this diet - it's tons of polyphenols (antioxidants), and vitamin E. adds to the various benefits of vegetable oil; studies have shown that it also increases the speed of fat oxidation.

In other words, it helps you burn fat more efficiently! Vegetable oil contains a comparatively sizable amount of calories, so moderation is the key to its use. Add vegetable oil to your daily diet. Yes, it's costlier but worthwhile.

Be careful; extra-calorie vegetable oil is 120 kilocalories per large tablespoon! So, if you begin using it, consume no more than one teaspoon per day, about 40 calories.

Eat Off the Plate

Do not eat directly from your bag: put the quantity of food you would like in a plate or bowl, and put the container away before eating. This tip will help you reduce the danger of returning for an additional serving (especially if you create access to the food container).

Be Flexible

Adhering to an excessively ordered and disciplined diet isn't very fun, and weight loss should be joyful. Once you believe what you get due to losing weight, you've got a real reason to smile. You'll make mistakes and sometimes believe why you're doing all this, but once you see and feel the result, you'll realize that each one of the difficulties was worthwhile. Rocky said better of all: "It doesn't matter what percentage times you strike, but it's important what percentage times you'll rise after a strike." the foremost important thing is to stick to the goal each day and luxuriate in it. Then you reach the goal before you think!

Say Goodbye to Sugar

Refined sugar and lots of artificial sweeteners are the enemies of weight loss (and health). A standard person eats a substantial amount of sugar! Things like sweets and cakes are practically barren of nutritional value and alienate you from healthy food -

you actually won't have a snack with fresh peas after you've got eaten the pie, right? The American Heart Association recommends that ladies should not consume more than six teaspoons of sugar per day (24 grams).

The matter is that it's hiding in places you do not even suspect (for now). Many where (from seasoning to crackers) - read the labels.

You can find a natural alternative. For instance, treat yourself to fruits, you'll try something healthy; a superb alternative to sugar for the load loss process is Stevia (sugar substitute).

Do Not snap at Others!

If you snap at pieces of food from plates of people (friends, children, spouse), then stop. All of those calories count, especially sweets. You'll bite here and there - very quickly, you'll eat as many calories as intended for your dinner, if less. Therefore, the number of those calories will always be underestimated because you probably did not eat from your plate. But it still matters a lot! Not only that, but most people also don't include such "little bits" in their food magazines. If you would like to share the dessert, cut it far away from your piece to count these calories.

Be Active at Work

Let's face it; most folks sit considerably in the working day. Attempt to take active breaks as often as possible: rise from the table and take a walk, ask your colleague's face to face, and not by email, go up the stairs! If you'll attempt to get a desktop for yourself that you simply will be standing at, not sitting at. Drive to figure every day?

Stand to burn excess calories. Remember, even small steps take into consideration.

Eat Nuts!

Nuts are full of healthy compounds, from healthy fats and antioxidants to valuable minerals and vitamins. Studies have shown that to reduce, eating large portions of wholesome food is way more critical than dieting yourself. Because simply put, you'll have less space in your stomach, and you'll not reach for unhealthy foods when your stomach is filled with healthy eating. Nuts are ideal in this sense because they contain an excessive amount of fiber and slowly digest. Also, healthy fats will assist you to feel full. Remember that we aren't talking about fried, salted nuts - buy natural nuts and take a couple with you for a walk to stay your hunger in check.

Keep an eye fixed on Your Weekend.

Most people can maintain a healthy and even strict diet during the workweek, but when the weekend comes, all efforts go nowhere! You want to be reliable, not weak, at the weekend. One of the items you'll do to make things easier is to permit yourself one relaxed meal every weekend.

That doesn't mean that you simply will come off to the fullest (or rather, "eat yourself") for an entire week of abstention from desserts! You'll not be so strict on yourself when choosing products for this meal. Be careful; don't let this relaxed meal become a relaxed day. Otherwise, you risk ruining all of your weekly work! Many of us don't even need such relaxation, so it all depends on your personal preferences.

Count Calories

Studies have shown that folks who count calories have significantly higher success in reducing and maintaining weight than those that don't. Counting also helps you structure your diet and detect unexpected high-calorie enemies!

Chapter 3

Advantages

Advantages You'll get a raise

It's outrageous, but really: your boss may treat you better when she loses weight. Consistent with a study in Health Economics, obese people, especially women, weigh about 2.5% their normal-weight than their colleagues. Although this might not sound astronomical, it's the difference between making $60,000 and $61,500 a year. Enough extra cash to travel on vacation or buy a gorgeous designer bag!

According to the newest reports from the University of Surrey and Oxford University, reducing a healthy weight may increase promotion probabilities. The psychologist behind the study found that weight and perceived attractiveness play an important role in whether someone will find the perfect job or get a promotion. They found that the heavier the person, the lower their chance. Things get worse: if you're overweight women, your career development opportunities are smaller than men.

You'll are talking about seasonal allergies for so long

If your eyes become itchy every spring after the flowers begin to bloom annually, it's going to be that your weight is affected. That's because overweight can damage the adrenal glands and system respiratory, exacerbating asthma, and allergy symptoms.

Now that you simply became slim, you'll be ready to abandon the inhaler and reduce the popping of seasonal pills, just without lecture the MD first! Do you still sniff after you've discarded the medicine? Eat this, not like that! Seasonal Bible to fight against spring allergies.

You'll Be ready to Throw medicine

You already know that reaching a healthy weight can prevent diseases like heart condition and diabetes, but does one understand that losing weight can improve the present condition's symptoms? meaning that you simply could also be ready to take lower doses of current medicines or stop taking specific medication altogether. (This will prevent tons of cash!) Please contact your MD to ascertain the thinner types he or she thinks you'll enjoy.

Your priority may change

Dannii Martin, the blogger behind Hungry Healthy Happy, lost 98 pounds in 18 months after her doctor informed her that her heart had developed a drag. She wrote in a blog titled "Weight loss changed me, I'm not an equivalent person": "My focus has changed. Going bent on drinks was once the main target of my life, but now my life is more balanced.

Now, my work focus includes work, food (sometimes food, mostly healthy food), spending time with my loved ones, exercising, and overall happiness; in fact, some parts of my character haven't changed. I'm different. I even have completely changed my life." If you encounter similar changes, please do not be shocked.

You'll Sleep Better

They seem entirely unrelated, but playing, sleeping, and weight loss have a replacement relationship. Apnea is usually caused by excess weight on the neck, and weight loss can disappear after only 5%. Therefore, after losing weight, you'll sleep better, which may help you reduce further. To make the foremost of your night sleep, checking this stuff before getting to bed can reduce weight

You'll Be More Relaxed

Fred Lechuga, who wrote the blog Fat 2 Fit Fred, once experienced terrible violence before dropping a powerful 150-pound thing. However, thanks to the load loss, he said he was cold, sort of a cucumber. He wrote in his book "Reducing Weight, Maintaining Weight: Life After Losing 100 Pounds": "When I used to be overweight, and behind the wheel, my finger was tons out of the window once I commuted. (I know, I know, this is often irrelevant.) Now, my attitude is like; "No matter what guy, cut me off, I do not care." A number of these could also be the results of maturity now, but I do believe that, thanks to lifestyle changes,

I'm just a more relaxed person." Although everyone responds differently to weight loss, leisurely people may only be thin and weak. one among the various privileges!

Your memory may improve

If remembering the names of individuals has been bothering you all of your life, then the additional weight you carry could also be blamed on you. In one study, women's memory test after losing weight was better than before losing weight. Why? Brain scans show that when these women reduce, they will have more activity once they make memories.

Activities in this memory will decrease, indicating that carrying an excessive amount of pressure may make it harder for the brain to figure effectively. To make sure that you can recall important information later in life, make sure to avoid using these high-fat foods, damaging your brain.

Your Risk of Cancer is going to be Lower

Although most people know that smoking and sun exposure increases the danger of cancer, few realize that obesity is also related to the disease. (Inflammation caused by obesity should condemn.) It's terrible news. The great news is that consistent with cancer research on postmenopausal women, only 5% of weight loss can reduce inflammation. Studies of morbidly obese men undergoing bariatric surgery have similar results. It seems like the rationale for celebrating these delicious weight loss smoothies!

You'll Not Be So Hungry

Although some dieters said they felt hungry after losing weight, Fatsecret member Deana Garcia wrote on the website's message board that after losing 25 pounds, she "eats less" and not "has been hungry" as before. If we're to guess, it's because she ate healthy food rich in nutrients like protein and fiber to reinforce satiety. If you follow an identical weight-loss strategy, you'll reduce hunger while reducing food intake and maintaining the trimmer's body.

You'll Spend extra money

According to the Health Affairs report, those who maintain a healthy weight spend 42% less on medical bills and health expenses than overweight. They save Benjamins; these scrawny little girls spend $1,429 less annually than big fools. There's extra money in the wallet, which is one more reason to make yourself slim.

Reddit user Oppiken said that his complexion was clear after losing weight, and his hair looked healthier and "less lily." Because many of the nutrients in healthy foods have cosmetic effects, it's safe to assume that his weight-loss diet may thank him for his improved appearance. Does one also want to reduce and improve complexion? Add these best skin-friendly foods to your weekly lineup.

You'll Sweat Less

When you are overweight, you wearing a heavier vest in a hot room 24/7 is not an easy task. (Fat can insulate the body and lift blood heat.) that's why obese people sweat more than slim people. Before losing weight, Reddit user, some bunny loves you, said her sweat stains were so severe that she had to travel to class a quarter-hour earlier to wipe herself in the bathroom with a wet towel. Since losing weight, she is happy to report that she is no longer super sweaty and "no longer worried about embracing others."

Chapter 4

Disadvantages

You'll Have Sagging Skin and Stretch Marks

Relaxation, sagging skin, and stretch marks are the results of losing weight too quickly. Malina Linkas Malkani, a registered nutritionist at a nutritionist, told INSIDER that this happened because the skin could not contract fast enough because of the physical body.

"The focus is on slow and stable weight loss, reducing about one to 2 pounds per week in order that the skin has time to shrink with the body."

She also recommends resistance exercises to stop the loss of lean muscle. Consistent with "Prevention," using sunscreen and using collagen-based serum or retinoids to create muscles can help prevent skin sagging and eating more produce in this weight loss.

When weight loss occurs quickly, and the skin is slack and limp, some people will choose surgery to get rid of it. It's worth noting that, consistent with the American Board of Aesthetic Surgery, the method will cause visible scars and take weeks to recover.

You'll Stop parturition

The pressure exerted on the body in this weight loss also can affect your period. When you are consistent with it, the more weight you lose, the faster you miss it; the more likely your period will be affected. Caroline Apovian, director of the middle for Nutrition and Weight Management at Boston center, explained that this happens because your body thinks it's hormonally hungry. She said to INSIDER: "Lectin will close the menstrual period because your body thinks it's hungry, and it's not healthy for the lady who was going hungry." "So, your body cannot save your menstrual period. So, you will not be pregnant and have a drag."

You'll feel cold

According to Apovian, this common weight loss complaint is said to your rate and hormone changes. Abovian said: "When losing weight, your body will reduce the speed of metabolism to save lots of energy." "And in terms of saving energy, it doesn't have too many calories to stay warm." One more reason you'll feel colder is that you simply do not have fat that acts as an insulator. This makes the report say that without an additional layer, your body will be more sensitive to temperature changes when losing weight.

You'll Not Be ready to nod off

The relationship between sleep and food is complicated. The National Broadcasting Corporation's "Better" reported that eating not only affects sleep but also affects your food choices. Consistent with the National Institute of Neurological Disorders and Stroke, the essential principle of sleep comes right down to a chemical called adenosine, which forms in your body before melatonin rises. Although we all know that rest is the key to successful dieting and weight loss, sleep could also be harder in this weight loss due to dietary changes.

Abovian said: "If you would like to urge an honest night's sleep, you would like your tryptophan levels to extend, and therefore the way to do that is to make the carbohydrate contain a little amount of protein, which increases the brain and melatonin Tryptophan levels." "When you're under-eating, or your calorie intake reduces, your hormone balance will change, so you will not be hooked in to sleeping. Instead, you'll be activated, and therefore the body is trying to find food."

Abovian said: "This isn't an act of obviating everything, but your interest in food is the hormones that it provides." "The ghrelin released in the stomach causes you to very hungry, and you'll find different foods more attractive."

The theory is supported by a study that found that the tastes of individuals who lost weight through bariatric surgery have changed. Consistent with a Time magazine report, almost 87% of patients reported this alteration after surgery, and half of them said the food tasted terrible. Those with dull taste buds lost more weight than their peers who claimed to possess enhanced taste. Consistent with "Health" magazine, that's because the hormonal changes affect how taste receptors transmit information to the brain.

You'll Have Difficulty Continuing to reduce

Weight loss and weight loss plateaus are common, usually due to reduced rates. Consistent with Malkani, this is often thanks to the loss of lean body mass, and therefore the body now requires fewer calories to figure. She said: "Don't fall under the trap of thinking that you simply can return to your previous eating habits after losing weight." "To maintain weight loss, you want to adopt a dietary change in your lifestyle, not a short-term diet."

Your relationship may change

If you and your partner are committed to a healthy lifestyle and don't let weight loss become a contest, making healthy changes and losing weight can benefit your relationship. However, if your partner doesn't make these changes with you, there could also be trouble in heaven. The matter is to try to adapt your partner to changes in your lifestyle once they are unwilling. Judith Baker, director of the Baker Institute for Cognitive Behavioral Therapy and author of "Baker Diet Solutions," said: "It's almost impossible to undertake or force someone to become healthier." "He knows he should exercise and eat less.". He doesn't want to. Otherwise, he will roll in the hay."

According to women's health, avoiding these problems boils right down to compromises in communication and relationships. Therefore, rather than spending tons of your time cooking together (which has its interpersonal advantages), it's better to check in for competition together with your partner to exercise. Find ways to be inclusive without having to impose on your partner.

Chapter 5

How to Stop Binge Eating and find a new Balance

Early life growth sets the stage for later development and can affect the susceptibility of individuals to disease. Early life growth should also be taken into account in the personalization of nutrition for mental health.

During the time of early brain development, any results of dietary intervention (the so-called first 1000 days, e.g. from conception to 2 years of age) may have a greater impact on later health than later life interventions. Increasing fundamental understanding of how nutrients influence signaling processes that are important for brain functions would also make progress.

Brains general functions: including those that act via the gut microbiota, such as metabolic, endocrine, and immune and other signaling processes.

The brain accounts for about 13 percent of lean body weight in newborn humans and its further growth and development is subject to both energy and nutritional constraints. Reliable access to a sufficient dietary supply is necessary during this time of rapid development. To date, the cognitive impairments triggered by early- life malnutrition have been a major focus in the field of nutritional psychiatry. Early-life diet has been shown to influence cognitive performance later in life in rodents and humans.

In addition, groups that are vulnerable at elevated risk of neurological impairment, such as preterm-born infants or small-term-born infants of gestational age, encourage a clear correlation between nutritional status and the risk of neurological impairment.

Although all nutrients are essential for brain growth, protein, iron, choline, folate, iodine, vitamins A, D, B6, and B12 and long-chain polyunsaturated fatty acids are key nutrients that help neuro development. Experimental studies have shown that the cyto- architecture of the cerebral cortex during fetal development can be irreversibly disrupted by iodine deficiency.

And it induces irregular migratory patterns of neurons that are associated with children with cognitive disability. Iron deficiency anemia during infancy has been shown to be associated with brain connectivity changes, but it has also been shown that the reverse has occurred. More subtle dietary changes may also influence the early development of the brain. Breast milk supplies lipids and, more precisely, omega-3 and 6 polyunsaturated fatty acids DHA (docosahexaenoic acid) and ARA (arachidonic acid), but their concentrations in breast milk are influenced by the mother's dietary intake.

Researchers using mice found that the absorption of omega-3 fatty acids into neuronal membranes was positively affected by a diet either enriched with omega-3 fatty acids or with reduced omega-6 fatty acid levels. Such a low omega-6 diet has also recently been shown to fully abolish cognitive impairments caused by early life stress in adult mice. A recent research has shown an increase in cognitive habits and plasticity markers in the adolescent brain in rats exposed to a diet supplemented with omega-3 polyunsaturated fatty acids, eicosapentaenoic acid, docosahexaenoic acid, and docosapentaenoic acid and vitamin A following psychological stress.

The long-term effects of early-life stress were alleviated by the dietary intervention of the milk fat globule membrane (MFGM) and the pre-biotic blend of poly-dextrose/galacto-oligo-saccharide using a rat maternal separation model.

These results illustrate the essential role of a healthy diet in providing a sufficient supply of nutrients to sustain brain growth for later cognitive function and the importance of early life development to (later) psychiatric disease susceptibility, which could explain, at least in part, the variability of treatment effects observed.

Chapter 6

The concept of food and Brain

The data highway of the brain, spinal cord, and nerves is like a telephone system that interacts with your digestive organs through your mind. Let's say that you're about to eat a cone

of ice cream. In the upper center of the brain-the cerebral cortex-the idea and picture of that ice cream exists. From there, data is electrochemically relayed to the limbic system, which is known to be the "lower" part of the brain. Emotions and main physiological functions such as starvation, hunger, temperature, sex drive, heart rate and blood pressure are regulated by the limbic system. A pea- sized set of tissues known as the hypothalamus is inside the limbic system, which combines the mind's actions with the body's biology.

In other words, it takes feedback from visual, emotional, and thought and translates this data into physiological responses. It's nothing short of a miracle here.

The hypothalamus can modulate this positive feedback by transmitting stimulation signals to the salivary glands, esophagus, stomach, intestines, pancreas, liver, and gallbladder through parasympathetic nerve fibers if the ice cream is your favorite flavor, say, chocolate, and you eat it with a full measure of delight. It will promote digestion and you will have a fuller metabolic breakdown of the ice cream while more effectively burning its calories.

The hypothalamus will take this negative feedback and send signals down the sympathetic fibers of the autonomic nervous system if you feel bad for eating the ice cream or judge yourself for eating it.

This initiates inhibitory responses in the digestive organs, ensuring that the ice cream will be consumed but not completely metabolized.

It may remain longer in your digestive system, which can decrease your healthy gut bacteria population and increase the release into the bloodstream of toxic by-products. In addition, through increased insulin and cortisol, inhibitory signals in the nervous system will decrease your calorie-burning power, which would cause you to store more of your guilt-infused ice cream as body fat. So, through the central nervous system, the thoughts you think about the food you consume immediately become reality in your body.

The brain does not discriminate between an actual stressor or an imaginary one. If you sat alone, happy and content in a room, and started thinking about the guy who did you wrong years ago, and if that story still holds a charge for you, your body will turn rapidly to the physiological stress-state-increased heart rate and blood pressure, followed by decreased digestive function.

The brain considers any guilt about food, shame about the body, or judgment about health to be stressors and is immediately transformed into its electro-chemical equivalents in the body. You can eat the healthiest meal on the planet, but the digestion of your food goes down and your fat storage metabolism will go up if you think of toxic thoughts. Similarly, you could consume a nutritionally challenged meal, but the nutritious power of your food would be enhanced if your head and heart are in the right position.

Let's take a fresh look at one of the most convincing phenomena in science to fully understand the influence of the mind over metabolism: the placebo effect. Here is my favorite instance of this remarkable force.

In 1983, a new chemotherapy treatment was being tested by medical researchers. The actual drug being tested was received by one group of cancer patients, while another group was given a placebo, a fake harmless, inert chemical substance.

As you might know, to assess the true efficacy, if any, of the substance in question, pharmaceutical companies are forced by law to test all potential products against a placebo. No one thought twice during the course of this study that 74 percent of cancer patients undergoing actual chemotherapy had one of the most common side effects of this treatment: losing their hair. However, quite remarkably, 31% of the placebo chemotherapy patients-an inert saltwater injection-also had an odd side effect: they also lost their hair. The power of expectation is such.

The only explanation why they lost their hair to those placebo patients is that they thought they would. They associated chemotherapy with going bald, like many individuals.

What do you think happens when we think to ourselves, "This cake is fattening, I really shouldn't be eating it," or "I'm going to eat this fried chicken, but I know it's bad for me," or "I enjoy eating my salad because it's really healthy?" if the influence of the mind is intense enough to make our hair fall out when taking a placebo. ”

It's definitely not saying that if we believe that it's good for us, we can eat poison without any harm. I say that what we believe about the material that we eat can have a powerful effect on how it affects the body. Millions of people eat and drink every day while thinking about their meals with clear and compelling feelings.

Consider some of the foods to which you have good links:

"Salt's going to increase my blood pressure." "Fat is going to make me fatter."

"Sugar is going to rot my teeth." "Without my cup of coffee, I can't make it through the day."

"This meat will raise my level of cholesterol." "My bones will build this calcium."

Some of these statements may be true to a certain degree. But is it possible that we are instigating these effects? And if these impacts are the inevitable product of eating these foods, do you see how, with the power of our expectations, we can change those outcomes?

Its type is very commonplace. Researchers have estimated that 35 to 45 percent of all prescription medicines can owe their efficacy to the power of placebo and that 67 percent of all over-the-counter medicines are also focused on placebo, such as headache remedies, cough medicines, and appetite suppressants. The placebo response in some studies is as high as 90 percent.

It is amazing that very few have made the apparent connection between placebo power and food in the scientific community. The placebo effect is, therefore, integrated into the nutritional process. On a day-to-day basis, it's intensely present every time we eat. It's like phoning to your own inner dietary pharmacy in a prescription.

What we assume, through nerve pathways, the endocrine system, the circulation of neuropeptides, the immune network, and the digestive tract, is alchemically translated into the body.

Chapter 7

The relationships between mental Health and food

Many individuals are attempting to use self-help to regain care of their mental health, and to find ways they can use alongside or even instead of prescription medicine. One

approach for self-help is to make improvements to what we consume, and there is a growing interest in how emotional and mental wellbeing can be influenced by food and nutrition.

Scientific evidence is emerging to support this, but scientists have several obstacles to address and, in the meantime, some medical practitioners remain unconvinced of the relation between food and mood. Nevertheless, the value of food and nutrition for preserving or enhancing their emotional and mental health is demonstrated by supportive feedback from people who have made improvements to their diet.

How mood is influenced by food?

The cause-and-effect relationship between food and mood has many theories. Some instances are the following:

Blood sugar level variations are correlated with mood and energy changes and are caused by what we eat.

Brain chemicals affect the way we think, sound and act (neurotransmitters, such as serotonin, dopamine and acetylcholine).

They might be influenced by what we have eaten.

Abnormal reactions, such as artificial colourings and flavourings, to artificial chemicals in foods may occur.

There are reactions that may be due to an enzyme deficiency necessary to digest a food. For example, lactase is required to digest lactose (milk sugar); without it, you can build up a milky intolerance.

Individuals may become food hypersensitive. This can cause what are known as food allergies or sensitivities that are delayed or concealed.

Mental wellbeing may be impaired by inadequate levels of vitamins, minerals and essential fatty acids, with certain symptoms associated with specific nutritional deficiencies. Relations between low levels of certain B-vitamins and symptoms of schizophrenia, low levels of mineral zinc and eating disorders, and low levels of omega-3 oils and depression have been shown, for instance.

Chapter 8

What is the Psychological Connection of Food & the Mind

Generally, it is agreed that how we feel will affect what we eat or drink (mood to food). What is less well understood is how our eating will impact our mental functioning (food to

mood). One example of what a dynamic relationship is the use of caffeine. Caffeine, present in tea, coffee, cola and chocolate beverages, is perhaps the world's most commonly used behavior-modifying substance. If we are feeling tired and irritable, we always prefer to drink it, because it can give us a lift and help us focus. There are also a number of positive psychological associations with enjoying a cup of coffee or tea. By sitting down with a cup of tea, we meet a friend for 'coffee and a chat' or giving ourselves a break, and these things are really important. But too much caffeine can cause symptoms, such as anxiety, nervousness and depression, (which is a different amount for each of us). Any diet and mood research needs to take this two-way relationship into account and involve the psychological factor behind what we want to consume.

It's well worth taking a look at what you are currently consuming and drinking before researching the particular foods that could affect your mental and emotional health. Typically, keeping a food and drink diary every day, for around one week, is the most effective way to do this. It seems to work better at the moment you have it, if you can write down what you eat and drink.

The more detail you provide in your journal, the more valuable it is going to be; the time and the average quantities you eat, for example, you should also write down. When they look back on what they have eaten, people are always shocked. An significant first step forward is greater understanding.

What To Look For Or Take Note Of In A Diet

A fundamental thing to consider for you would be: is there any food or form of food I eat almost every day or in particularly large quantities? The foundation of a balanced diet is to maintain a balance between a wide range of foods, where over a period of days the variety is spread out. Some foods are consumed by most individuals on most days, possibly because they are commonly considered safe to consume. Unfortunately, these may be the very foods that affect your health with a hidden, but crippling, impact.

It is always a mixture of consuming too much of certain foods and not enough of others that leads to symptoms such as anxiety or depression. An important part of making adjustments to your diet is ensuring that you do not go on a regular basis without the nutrients your body needs. So, if you cut back on one meal, instead of that, you would typically need to replace anything close to eating. For example, this can mean substituting wheat-based bread for bread made from rye flour.

Foods That Affects The Mood

While the exact cause-and-effect relationship between different foods and moods has yet to be fully understood, many people have found that they can relate certain foods to how they feel by eating (or not eating). Alcohol, sugar, caffeine, chocolate, wheat (such as bread, cookies, and cakes), dairy products (such as cheese), certain artificial additives (or E numbers) and hydrogenated fats are among the foods and beverages that most frequently trigger problems.

Other foods that are widely consumed, such as yeast, maize, eggs, oranges, soy and tomatoes, may also cause symptoms in some people. Important improvements in a wide variety of mental health conditions will result from changes in what we eat. The following changes have been reported: mood fluctuations, anxiety, panic attacks, cravings or food addictions, depression (including postnatal depression), irritable or violent feelings, focus, memory issues, premenstrual syndrome (PMS), obsessive-compulsive feelings, eating disorders, psychotic episodes, sleeplessness, exhaustion, behavioral and learning disorders, and se (SAD).

In order to feel healthy, which foods you need to eat?

For a balanced mind and body, water is the most vital material. It is easy to miss drinking the necessary six to eight glasses a day, which is a low-cost, convenient, self-help measure that can improve how we feel, both mentally and physically, easily.

The nutrients required to nourish the mind and body are given by consuming at least five daily portions of fresh fruit and vegetables (organically grown, if possible). (One part equals a handful or so.)

It's best not to miss breakfast, keep your meals on a regular basis, and choose foods that slowly release energy, including oats and unrefined whole grains. Some protein foods, such as beef, fish, beans, eggs, cheese, nuts or seeds, are also essential to eat every day.

These eating habits, as well as supplying nutrients, help reduce the adverse effects of fluctuating levels of blood sugar, including irritability, low concentration, exhaustion, depression, and cravings for food. For the development and healthy functioning of the brain, essential fatty acids, especially the omega-3 type found in oil-rich fish such as mackerel and sardines, linseeds (flax), hemp seeds and their oils, are vital.

There are also major 'good mood' nutrients in other seeds and nuts, such as sunflower seeds, pumpkin seeds, brazil nuts and walnuts.

An example of putting these guidelines into effect is The Mind Meal. To draw attention to the essential relationship between food and mood, this was launched by Mind. It shows what can be achieved for emotional and mental health with some of the positive mood foods commonly recommended as beneficial. Information about the Mind Meal and other nutritious recipes and foods is available under 'Treatments' in the 'How can we help you' section of Mind's website.

How To Go About Changing A Diet

If you start by making improvements slowly, one at a time, and only for a trial period, it is probably a lot easier. It takes a bit of effort and time to change what you eat; trying out new and different foods can mean you need to shop in new places. Hopefully, you're going to enjoy making these improvements and find them a positive experience.

Smaller improvements, implemented one at a time, should you find them helpful, are easier to handle and keep up. If you make more than one shift at a time, you're not going to be able to tell what an impact is having. Some modifications can even be unnecessary, but once you try, you won't know.

It is possible to extend this step-by- step approach later, and it could be helpful to maintain a food and mood diary.

Sometimes, just for the first few days, a shift in the diet causes some unwanted side effects. For example, if people suddenly stop drinking coffee, they can get signs of withdrawal, such as headaches, which then begin to clear up after a few days, when they begin to feel much better. If you cut down gradually, as if you were weaning yourself from a medication, symptoms such as these can be minimized. There are, clearly, certain costs associated with making improvements to what you consume, but they can be rewarded by substantial mental and physical health benefits.

Supplements and Nutritional Information

A healthy and varied diet of health-supporting foods is the best source of vitamins and minerals; however, you might need to

With extra nutrients, supplement your diet. It is necessary to balance the different vitamins and minerals properly, and to avoid taking any nutrients in excess. Nutritional therapists are qualified to advise on

the use of supplements and can prescribe safe supplementation levels for individual needs.

Many people profit from taking a good-quality multivitamin and mineral supplement if it is not possible to get this support. It is also helpful to periodically take a fish oil supplement or a vegetarian oil mix containing 'omega-3' oils. Nutritional supplements are sold by health food stores, pharmacists and supermarkets. You might get a prescription for others.

Food Interaction With Medications

Some people want to try herbal alternatives that can help with the symptoms of depression, such as Hypericuum perforatium. However, if you are already taking any medication, prior to trying herbal remedies, it is important that you consult your doctor for guidance: some may interact with other medicines, stop them working, or cause additional adverse effects.

Note: it is very unwise to stop suddenly taking any medication that you have already prescribed. As they don't suit everybody, it's also worth consulting a medical herbalist about using these herbs.

In certain foods, antidepressants can interact with a naturally occurring substance called tyramine. A harmful increase in blood pressure can be caused by this, which can be indicated by a throbbing headache. Beans, yeast extract, meat extract, most cheeses, fermented soya bean extract and salted, smoked or pickled fish include foods containing particularly high levels of tyramine (especially pickled herring).

If you take MAOIs, you should avoid stale food or food that may be 'going off' because the action of bacteria on protein produces tyramine. This is especially relevant in the case of foods rich in protein, such as meat, fish or chicken. Stop game meats entirely. You can obtain a complete list from your doctor, dietitian or nutritional therapist of tyramine-containing foods.

Food Tests On Allergies Generally

If you have any classic food allergies, you will probably already know, because the symptoms will be quite fast and probably very dramatic. It is likely, however, to have certain delayed or secret food allergies or sensitivities that are less apparent, but may be harmful to your health, nevertheless.

The good news is that this form of allergy can be changed and does not need to be a serious or life-long illness, unlike classic food allergies, which tend to remain.

Food associated with delayed or hidden allergies or sensitivities is unlikely to be detected by tests for classic food allergies. Private monitoring for allergies can do so, but this is also costly. Another choice is a special diet called the diet of reduction and challenge.

This is when you completely cut out a food (elimination stage) for about two weeks and then reintroduce it (challenge stage).

A strong reaction to a food you have avoided confirms the dislike of that food by the body, and may also be used to diagnose sensitivities to food. With the support of a healthcare professional who is experienced in elimination diets, this method is almost certainly best tackled, who will be able to advise you on the full range of foods you will need to avoid and replace.

A rotation diet can be advised, where you consume different foods on different days.

During the phase of elimination, as you give your body a long rest from a meal, you may go through a phase of withdrawal and experience some unpleasant, but bearable, discomfort. You're then going to be in a state of increased sensitivity to the food.

You can have an exaggerated reaction to it if you eat it (either on purpose or accidentally), which some people find difficult to cope with. An experienced professional in the healthcare sector will be able to

In order to provide vital feedback on these aspects. It is possible to have a delayed answer to a food challenge as well.

This is when signs that present themselves just several hours later are induced by the food. If you are not aware of this possibility, then it is simple to miss them or not to connect them with the possibility.

Watch out for the food that you are eating again and again; this is where there will be invaluable clinical support. Indeed, before making any major changes to your diet, it is recommended that you consult a healthcare professional.

Chapter 9

Mindful Eating Practices

Mindful eating is a life skill that can lead individuals to enjoy a rewarding, safe and enjoyable relationship with food that is easy to understand. It is an ability that can help

individuals break free of 'food rules' and start embracing safe, versatile and comfortable eating habits.

Cautious eating is not a diet. Mindful eating refers to how we consume, not what we eat.

What is Mindful Eating?

It is about concentrating your attention and consciousness on the present moment to help detach from normal, unsatisfactory and unhealthy behaviors and habits to be conscious.

Eating with Mindfulness,

Put clearly, it's the opposite of eating mindlessly.

The mindful eating approach uses techniques that can help alter, both physically and emotionally, the way we react to food. Adopting a mentality of conscientious eating includes:

Being aware of the optimistic and nurturing possibilities of preparing and consuming food

By using the senses to discover, savour and taste, preferring to eat food that is both good and nourishing to the body Acknowledging reactions without judgment to food

Being mindful of the signs of physical hunger and satiety to direct decisions to start and stop eating

Identify personal causes, including emotions, social expectations or certain foods, for mindless eating.

Why attempt meticulous eating?

Research shows that mindful eating can help individuals regulate binge eating and overeating, enjoy eating, and feel more in contact with the internal appetite and sacrifice signals of the body.

A lot of us might not be conscious of the reasons why we eat mindlessly. Some common contributors may be:

Not understanding the difference between eating with and without hunger;

Don't stop listening to what you are told by your body signals; Confusing hunger and thirst

Allowing yourself to get hungry and/or to eat too easily

Eat an amount that should make you feel complete, but not satisfied.

Eating at a later stage in case you get hungry

In response to some feelings, eating to relieve a state of mind, such as tiredness or boredom.

The mindful eating strategy uses approaches that promote awareness of the senses while eating to bring you into the present moment. These techniques include: keeping a careful log, slowing down while eating, concentrating on eating (not watching TV or reading), and shopping and preparing food consciously.

Mindless eating is prevalent because we are conditioned to eat from a very early age in response to external signals (time of day, availability of certain foods, for convenience, to relieve boredom, out of habit, to clear our plate, as a reward) rather than in response to hunger.

Mindful Eating Strategies

Mindful eating strategies can help decrease the risk of binge eating. These include:

1. Every 2-3 hours, consume small or moderate amounts of food.

2. Asking a few fundamental questions before eating

Am I starving? Am I thirsty? What sort of food/drink do I like, if so?

3. Set up a nice place to eat and neatly arrange food on your plate. Don't eat while walking or standing!

4. Being in the present before starting to feed (3 deep breaths)

5. Eat slowly, paying attention to the food's odor, taste, tone, texture and appearance.

6. In between mouthfuls, bring utensils or food down.

7. Checking in with your hunger signals every few minutes

8. If you are still hungry, stop eating just before you feel satisfied and wait 10-20 minutes before consuming more food.

9. Enjoy the meal. You will never be happy if you do not like food.

You may also like to pursue journaling, which is a discipline focused on mindfulness. You should use a journaling system or methodology that suits you and that over a long period of time is sustainable.

Some people like to carry a notebook or journal around with them; before they go to bed, some people keep a journal to write in. Others keep their machine with a food diary or notes. It could be a list of foods you ate, a poem, a summary of your feelings or a painting. It doesn't really matter what you write.

Yoga, meditation and walking meditation are also exercises that you would like to try based on mindfulness.

Here is an easy mindful eating exercise that you can do to practice the ability of mindfully eating at home.

1. Choose one food piece. It could be a raisin, a mandarin slice, a cookie or a potato chip.

2. Begin by taking a look at the food. Test the shape, color and texture.

3. Bring the food to your nose and smell it.

4. Place it on your tongue with the food. Note how your salivary glands respond.

5. Be mindful of the sounds in your mouth and the feel of your tongue. Take a taste.

6. Note how the food's texture varies when you chew.

7. Swallow it now; as the food moves down your throat to your stomach, pay attention.

8. Now tell quietly to yourself the name of the meal.

9. At least once each meal, try to practice a thoughtful slice.

Through the limited success of simplistic models in genetics and neuroscience in describing and predicting eating behavior in humans, the need for a detailed explanation of eating behavior has become important. In conjunction with the effectiveness of therapies that normalize eating styles in obesity and eating disorders, the lack of cognitive approaches reveals the central role of eating in coping with these issues.

Women have been found to eat at either a decelerated or constant pace in the continuous recording of eating activity and satiety over the course of a meal. Unlike decelerated eaters, linear eaters are unable to regulate their food consumption when the rate of eating is experimentally increased or decreased and their level of satiety is disassociated from the actual intake of food.

Their reactions to these experimental challenges simulate anorexic and binge eating disorder patients' eating habits and satiation ratings.

The general developments of an improved approach for single meal analysis, which incorporates video derived and intake data, enables the analysis over time of the different behavioral components of the meal. In order to compare eating habits between different groups of people, semi-automation, high validity and reliability make this technique perfect. In decelerated and linear eaters, the chewing duration, the chewing distribution within the chewing sequences, and the pauses between mouthfuls remain constant throughout the meal.

The total weights of the mouth full of food decreases and in the decelerated eaters, but not the linear ones, the length of the chewing sequences increases over time, demonstrating the essence of deceleration.

In addition, the default chewing frequency, quantified by the use of chewing gum, is less linear than that of decelerated eaters, suggesting that there is a baseline disparity between the two classes in the default chewing frequency.

Linear eating is suggested to be a behavioral risk factor for the development of disordered eating, and although repetitive disordered eating is the cause of eating disorders, it is suspected that the accompanying chewing characteristics may be the mediator of the emotional profile that characterizes eating disorder patients.

The result of eating disorders remains poor and there is little, if any impact, on widely used treatment strategies. This situation is suggested to have occurred because of the inability to understand that patients with eating disorder symptoms are epiphenomena of hunger and the resulting disordered eating. Humans have evolved to cope with the hunger challenge and anatomically flexible neuroendocrine systems that have been under this evolutionary strain are exhibiting synaptic plasticity to allow flexibility.

So many of the neuroendocrine general changes in hunger are reactions to the externally imposed food scarcity, and the associated neuroendocrine secretions promote, as required, behavioral adaptation rather than simply making a person consume more or less food. It provides a parsimonious, neuro-biologically realistic description of why eating disorders are emerging and why they are retained. It is suggested that when food intake is reduced, the brain mechanisms of reward are activated and that disordered eating behavior is subsequently maintained by conditioning to the circumstances in which the disordered eating behavior developed for attention through the neural system. Patients are taught how to eat normally, their physical activity is controlled, and external heat is given to them in a method based on this framework. In a randomized controlled trial, the method has been proven efficient.

Chapter 10

Eating Disorders and Problems

An eating issue is any relationship you find challenging with food.

In our lives, food plays an important role and most of us spend time worrying about what we consume. We can often try to eat healthier, have cravings, eat more than normal, or lose our appetite. It is natural to change your eating habits every now and then.

But if it feels like food and eating is taking over your life, then it can become a problem.

A lot of people believe that you would be over- or underweight if you have an eating disorder, and that having a certain weight is often correlated with a particular eating problem. It's a myth here. Eating disorders can affect anyone, irrespective of age, gender or weight.

If you have an issue with food, you might:

Limit the amount of food you consume

When eating, you eat more than you need or feel out of control.
Eat a lot secretly

Feeling really concerned about eating or digesting food

In response to challenging feelings (when you don't feel physically hungry), eat plenty of food.

Eat only certain kinds of food or adhere to a strict set of diet guidelines and feel very nervous and disappointed if you have to eat something different.

Doing stuff to get rid of what you eat (purging)

Stick to strict guidelines on what you can and can't consume and how food should taste and get really offended if you violate those rules.

The thought of eating such foods is widely disliked. Eat stuff that isn't even food

Be fearful of those forms of food or public eating Dream about food and eating a lot or all the time.

Compare your body with others and care a lot about their shape or size.

Check, check and weigh a lot of your body and base your self-worth on how much you weigh or whether your checks and tests are passed.

Difference Between Eating Disorder And Eating Problems

A medical diagnosis based on your dietary habits and medical testing on your weight, blood and body mass index is an eating disorder (BMI).

An eating issue is any relationship you find challenging with food. This can be just as painful as a diagnosed eating disorder to deal with.

How can your life be affected by eating problems?

Problems with eating are not just about food. They can be about daunting stuff and painful emotions that you can find difficult to convey, face or overcome. A way to hide these issues, even from yourself, may be to concentrate on food.

Eating issues can impact you in many ways.

Maybe you:

It's hard to focus and feel very tired

Discover the food or food management has become the most important thing in your life.

Feeling depressed and worried

Feeling embarrassed or guilty and fearful of other individuals finding out

Feel isolated from friends or relatives who don't know how you feel or who are angry and disappointed that they can't do anything to help you

Prohibit social events, dates and restaurants or public eating It's difficult to be spontaneous, fly or go somewhere new.

Discover that your looks have changed

Discover that other individuals comment on your appearance in ways that you find difficult

You're bullied or teased about feeding and eating food. Build short- or long-term physical health concerns

You have to drop out of school or college, quit work or stop doing things that you love.

You can find that other individuals focus a lot on the impact that eating disorders may have on your body, or that they just think you have a problem if your body looks different from how they think it should be, and they don't really understand how difficult things are for you.

You may also have eating disorders and keep them secret, often for a very long time. You may not even be convinced that your diet and eating problems are a 'problem,' as it may feel like just a part of your daily life. Some individuals do not seek treatment because they feel that their problem is not serious enough or that their eating problem is not 'healthy enough'.

But it is okay to seek treatment if your relationship with food and nutrition impacts your life. No matter how much you weigh or what your body looks like, it does not matter.

Mental health conditions, such as depression, anxiety or obsessive-compulsive disorders, are often present in many people with eating problems. Food is one of the ways

by which it is possible to communicate anxiety, depression or obsessive-compulsive behaviors. An anxiety disorder associated with body perception, which can also lead to eating disorders, is body dysmorphic disorder.

What Eating Disorders Are

A medical diagnosis based on your dietary habits and medical testing on your weight, blood and body mass index is an eating disorder (BMI). This segment lists prevalent eating disorders and other diagnoses of disordered eating.

Nervosa bulimia Nervosa anorexia Eating Binge Condition

Another feeding or eating disorder specified (OSFED) Other diagnoses that apply to eating disorders

Food is one of the many ways by which our feelings and anxiety can be conveyed, so you may have a very complicated relationship with food that affects your mental health, but does not fall into any of the existing diagnostic categories. More than one eating disorder can also be experienced, or certain signs from each disorder can be experienced.

If you are eating problems are not easy for your doctor to categorize, they will not give you a particular diagnosis. But you might find it useful to consider some of the emotions and habits that can be correlated with particular eating disorders, even if you don't have a diagnosis, or choose to think about your experiences in a non- medical way.

Bulimia Nervosa-One

You may find that you consume large quantities of food in one go if you experience bulimia, because you feel irritated or worried (binging). After binging, you can then feel guilty or embarrassed and want to get rid of the food you have consumed (purging).

What you may be feeling:

Embarrassed and guilty

That your body is despised or that you are overweight Scared of being found out by friends and family Anxious or depressed

Lonely, particularly if no one knows about your issues with eating Quite low and furious, very tiny

When your mood changes rapidly or unexpectedly,

Just like you're caught in a loop of feeling out of control and trying to regain control.

Numb, as if emotions from bingeing or purging are blocked out.

What you may be doing:

Eat plenty of meals in one go (binge)

Go through eating stages,feeling guilty, purging, feeling hungry, and again eating

The whole day

When you binge, you eat food that you believe is bad for you. Hunger for yourself between binges

Eat secretly

Longing for those kinds of food

By getting yourself ill, using laxatives or exercising excessively, try to get rid of food that you have consumed (purge).

What could be going on with your body:

You can stay at the same weight, or you can also go from being overweight to being underweight.

You could be dehydrated, resulting in bad skin.

Your cycles could become erratic or stop entirely if you menstruate.

Your stomach acid will damage your teeth if you get sick and you can get a sore throat.

If you use laxatives, you can develop elongated irritable bowel syndrome (IBS)

Bowel disorder, constipation and heart disease

Nervosa Anorexia-Two

This is because you are not eating enough food to get the nutrition you need to stay healthy if you get an anorexia diagnosis. Often people believe that slimming and dieting are all about anorexia, but it's much more than that. It is also related at its heart to very low self- esteem, negative self-image and extreme feelings of distress.

What you may be feeling:

Like you can't think of anything but food Like you want to vanish,

That you must be perfect, perfect,

Like you're never good enough, never good enough,

Lonely, particularly if no one knows about your issues with eating

That you lose control by feeding, that you like you need to That you're hiding stuff from your friends and family

It's not just that you are overweight, and your weight loss Really afraid of putting weight on

Angry if someone is questioning you Tired and uninterested in stuff Depressed or suffering from suicide Anxious

What you may be doing:

Decrease food intake or fully quit eating

Count all the food's calories and spend a lot of time worrying about them.

Hide the food or throw it away secretly.

Prevent unhealthy foods, such as those with significant quantities of calories or fat, Read recipe books and cook elaborate meals for individuals, but do not eat them yourself.

Use medicines that claim to lower your appetite or speed up your digestion Consider losing weight all the time, Act a lot and have strict regulations about how much you need to do.

Making food laws, such as listing 'healthy' and 'bad' foods or consuming only items that are a certain color.

Establish very organized times for eating Check your body all the time and weigh it.

What could be going on with your body:

You may weigh less than you should or you may lose weight very easily,

You may become underdeveloped physically (in particular if anorexia starts before puberty)

You can feel insecure and move slowly, You could feel really cold the whole time,

Your cycles could become erratic or stop entirely if you menstruate. Your hair can become thin or fall out.

You may grow fine fluffy hair (called 'lanugo') on your arms and face, you may lose interest in sex or you may not be able to have or enjoy it.

You could find it difficult to focus.

Your bones can become brittle and conditions like osteoporosis can arise.

Disorder Of Binge Eating-Three

If you have a binge eating disorder, even if you want to, you may feel like you can't stop eating. Sometimes it is described as eating compulsively. If you have a binge eating disorder, you can rely on food to make you feel better or to conceal difficult emotions.

What you may be feeling:

Out of sight and as if you were unable to stop eating Ashamed or humiliated

Lonely and vacant

Highly poor, even useless, Dissatisfied with your body Anxious and stressed.

What you may be doing:

Choose meals all day, eat huge quantities all at once (bingeing) Eat without really thinking about it, especially when you do other stuff.

Consuming unhealthy foods daily

When you feel nervous, angry, bored or sad, eat for comfort. Hide the amount you consume

Eat until you feel sick or uncomfortably full Try a diet but find it challenging.

What could be going on with your body:

Maybe you should put on weight, You may experience health issues related to being overweight, such as diabetes, high blood pressure or joint and muscle pain.

You can feel breathlessness. Maybe a lot of you feel sick?

Sugar highs and crashes (having energy bursts followed by feeling very tired) can occur.

You may experience health problems like acid reflux and irritable bowel syndrome (IBS).

Other Defined Disorder Of Feeding And Eating Disorder

A condition that is becoming more prevalent is OSFED. You may have been diagnosed with an eating disorder not otherwise defined (EDNOS) in the past, but it is generally no longer used.

It means that you have an eating disorder if you are given an OSFED diagnosis, but you do not follow all the criteria for a diagnosis of anorexia, bulimia or binge eating disorder.

This does not indicate that the eating disorder is less serious, it only implies that it does not fall into existing categories of diagnosis. You can encounter any of the attitudes, emotions

Changes in the body and linked to other eating disorders.

Having an OSFED diagnosis will allow you to access counseling and support.

Some diagnoses associated with eating disorders:

Illness of rumination: You will frequently regurgitate your food if you have a rumination disorder (but you do not have a physical health problem to explain it). The food you regurgitate may be rechewed, re-swallowed or spat out.

Picaa: When you have pica, you can eat items that are not food on a daily basis and have little nutritional value (for example chalk, metal or paint). This could potentially be very detrimental.

Avoidant/restrictive condition of food consumption: You will feel a very strong desire to avoid food in general or certain foods due to their smell, taste or texture if you have ARFID. Anxiety will fill you with the thought of food. ARFID does not appear to be related to body image problems-it is an anxiety about the eating process itself.

What causes problems with eating?

There is no single source of problems with eating, with most experts assuming they come from a Combination of biological and environmental variables. It may be difficult to understand why it is For you, it has become a concern, as the reasons can be complex and confounding.

This segment encompasses:

Patterns and characteristics Challenging experiences of life Family problems

Social pressure

Physical and mental health challenges Biological and genetic variables Causes or moments 'at risk'

Traits And Habits

Individuals with eating disorders also share similar characteristics that can make them more

Vulnerable, such as:

Perfectionism-wanting to be perfect and rarely happy with what you've done.

Becoming really self-critical Being highly successful

Obsessive or compulsive behavior

A lack of confidence in expressing yourself.

Difficult Events in General

It is possible to relate the beginning of eating disorders to a traumatic event or trauma. Physical, emotional or sexual assault, the death of someone close to you, divorce, or severe family issues may all mean this. Or it may be school or career pressures, such as facing tests or being bullied.

When you go through big life changes, such as puberty, going to a new school, finding out your sexuality, or leaving home for the first time, eating problems also grow at the same time.

Issues From Family

Eating disorders may be exacerbated by childhood experiences or made worse. For instance, you could have started to use food as a way to gain more control over your life if your parents were especially strict, or home didn't feel like a healthy or consistent place. You could have established personality characteristics such as perfectionism and self-criticism if they have very high expectations of you, which may make you susceptible to eating issues.

And whether you were dieting, over-eating or having an eating disorder with other individuals in your family, this might have had an effect on you too.

Pressure From Social Peers

While there are definitely no eating disorders caused by social and cultural stresses, they can lead to them and help keep them going. Movies, magazines, social media, advertisements

And peer pressure means that signals about our bodies and our bodies surround us.

Ideas on how we should look (unachievable). You may not even realize that it is happening, but you may find yourself comparing yourself to these unrealistic images and, as a result, feeling bad about yourself. This kind of social pressure can make you feel like you're not good enough, which can have an effect on your self-esteem and body image.

Mental And Physical Challenges

You can also develop eating disorders if you have physical or mental health problems. It can make you feel powerless to have a physical health condition, so you can use eating or exercising as a way of feeling in control.

As you encounter a mental health condition such as depression, anxiety, bipolar disorder or body dysmorphic disorder, eating problems may begin. Emotions of low self-esteem, worthlessness or powerlessness may be related to them. Having an eating disorder will also lead you to experience these forms of problems with mental health.

Biological Influences And Genetics

Research has shown that your genes can influence whether you are vulnerable to an eating problem that develops.

It has also been found that there appear to be different concentrations of brain chemicals that regulate hunger, appetite and digestion in certain people with eating disorders. For instance:

Having too much or too little chemical serotonin in the brain can influence your mood and appetite.

Some individuals may be more responsive to the hormones that regulate hunger and fullness. This could make them more likely to binge or overeat.

There is ongoing study to find out more about the potential biological and genetic causes of issues with eating.

Triggers Or Causes

Any things could help to keep it going after it has grown, but not the cause of your eating habit.

If you have had eating issues in the past, or are currently struggling with recovery, you might find it helpful to think about factors that may make your eating problems more likely to come back, such as stressful conditions or going on a diet. These are considered 'triggers' or 'at risk' moments by certain people.

How You Can Help Yourself

It is very difficult to live with and heal from eating issues. You have to think about food on a regular basis and live in a changing body. But there are also ways you can support yourself to deal with these difficulties. This segment encompasses:

Speaking to individuals you trust Coping with incorrect principles Looking for peer assistance Handling relapses

Coping with the comments of others Coping with weight-putting

Change unhealthy habits

Cope with tough times of the year Remaining safe online

Am I able to think in terms of recovery?

For different people, healing means different things. It could mean that you never have to worry or act again about an eating disorder. Or it may mean that you still have them, but they don't happen as much and have less effect on your life.

Your views can also shift over time on how you view your relationship with food, and whether you want to recover. You may often feel like you don't have a problem, or that your behavior is very helpful to you. Your issue with eating can feel soothing, safe, or even exhilarating. And you may feel terrified of the changes that come with healing. For instance, you might feel:

Fear of weight loss or putting on Nervous to lose power

The problem of eating is so big a part of your life that you are not sure who you are without it.

It can take a long time to get there, whatever healing looks like to you, even though you feel ready to try. In years rather than weeks and months, you will have to remember. If you've tried to heal before, or have relapsed, you might begin to feel like you're totally out of support. However, even though it takes a long time, it is possible to feel better.

Talking to individuals you trust

Eating disorders, for many reasons, can be very hard to speak about. But even though people around you may find it difficult to understand eating issues, they will generally try to help as best as they can.

If you find it difficult to speak, you may try to write down stuff. For example, some people think that writing stuff in a letter will help get ideas out more clearly. You might also find it useful to present our data about eating issues to people to help them learn more about them.

Treating Myths and Misconceptions

If you are a male or an older woman, it's more difficult to talk about your experiences. But there are still eating problems for a lot of men and older women.

You will also find that your body changes more rapidly than your mental health. You may feel worse when you start to look healthier. When you are still still finding stuff really hard, other people might think you are recovered. It will help to keep up the conversation about how you feel, with people you trust.

Handling Deteriorations

Going back to old thoughts and behaviors is very common, especially around times when you are very stressed. It may be useful to recognize periods when you might be more at risk of returning to your eating habits. They may be:

Pregnancy and after birth

High stress cases such as examinations, marriage/civil union, break-up or moving home.

Think about the symptoms of early warning and what you can do to help stop things from getting worse. Signs of early warning may be:

Eating too little or too much

Negotiating over food and eating by yourself The need to purge

Fixing and worrying about food all the time Check your body or measure yourself more.

In their rehabilitation, most individuals may have failures. But after every failure, you may find that you understand more about yourself and your problem with eating. As part of a long, but achievable, process of improvement, it's necessary to try to be gentle with yourself and accept relapses.

Dealing with the comments of others

Many people don't realize what it's like to have a problem with eating. Some individuals can feel that commenting on your body, your weight, or how much (and what) you eat is okay.

They might think they're saying something good without understanding that you may find it hard to hear. This can be really hard to cope with.

For everyone, what helps or hurts is different. Trying to explain to family and family will help. Talking to friends on how you feel and what a more helpful or supportive response would be. But it's not always possible to stop people doing unhelpful stuff. It might be a good idea to think about how you're going to handle the stuff people might say.

Temporary Dealing With Weight Putting-On Or Gain

Recovery is not going to mean taking on weight for anyone. But this is an unbelievably daunting obstacle for certain individuals to deal with. Some individuals discovered that these tips worked for them:

Writing down the reasons why you want to rebound when things feel complicated, and look at them.

Take all of your clothes that do not suit or sell them online to a charity shop. Give yourself some fresh clothes in sizes that you feel secure in.

Try not to waste too much time staring at your body in mirrors or analyzing it.

If possible, stop measuring yourself.

Write down all of the healthy physical changes in your body that are occurring.

Have a rant or share your thoughts with someone who knows. Speak to other individuals.

Try not to make comparisons or waste too much time looking at photographs in magazines or online of people.

Dealing With Tough Times Of The Year

Some times of year may cause difficult thoughts and behaviors. Many times, these are gatherings that, including Christmas and birthdays, tend to revolve around food and eating with others.

Chat about how you feel and what will make things better with someone you trust.

Find different ways of celebrating, if possible.

Think of things that you can do to look after yourself when you find things challenging.

Understand and agree that there can be moments when you feel out of reach.

Be patient with yourself and don't set your goals too high.

Difficulties Of Feeding During Ramadan

You can find that Ramadan creates contradictions between your religion and your issues with eating and recovery if you are Muslim. Some people discover that fasting affects their eating problem- related thoughts and behaviors, especially if they are praised for eating very little. Others learn that iftar makes them feel out of control when dining with family and friends.

If you have a medical condition, although you may be excused from fasting, this may make you feel guilty. Other people might not know why you don't fast.

How To Stay Safe Online

You may find that you spend a lot of time comparing your body to other people especially if you have an eating disorder, often without really even realizing you are doing it. Pictures and photos always surround us, particularly on social media.

Be careful of how you feel when you're online and change the sites you visit and the people you follow if you need to. Taking a break from social media or changing your lifestyle is okay, because it plays less of a role in how you spend your time.

Note that many photographs have been tampered with to make the person look different. And images may have been filtered or photoshopped on social media.

Think of how you treat photos of yourself. Do they make you feel bad or do you feel you need to change them to hide how you really look?

Think about whether you're following someone whose videos make you feel bad or cause disturbing thoughts. Unfollow them if you can.

Block or prevent any websites promoting eating disorders.

Look for positive communities around food, recovery and positivity of the body.

What is the available treatment?

Treatment will help you develop balanced and healthier eating habits and help you face the underlying conditions that can cause your eating disorder and deal with it. This segment encompasses:

Speaking to the doctor

Free programmes for self-help Therapies for Conversation Medicine

Admission to a medical clinic

Techniques of non-invasive brain stimulation

Speaking To Your Physician

It can be frightening to talk about your eating issues, but if you want help and support, your first move is generally to see your doctor (GP). They should be able to refer you to further resources for specialists.

Self-Help Programmes Online

If you are diagnosed with bulimia or binge eating disorder, or if your eating disorders have similar symptoms, you can initially obtain assistance via an online self-help program.

Alongside the programme, you can receive brief support sessions. These could be over the phone or face-to-face. If you find it difficult to complete, or do not find it helpful, ask for more support from your GP.

Speaking About Treatments

The National Institute for Health and Care Excellence (NICE), which establishes health care best practice recommendations, suggests the following talking therapies for eating problems:

Cognitive behavioral treatment for eating disorders (CBT-ED). This is a specially modified type of CBT for the treatment of eating disorders, including anorexia.

Alternative forms of CBT occur for bulimia nervosa and binge eating disorder (CBT-BN) (CBT-BED).

Up to 40 treatments can be given for anorexia, with twice-weekly sessions during the first two or three weeks. You should be offered at least 20 sessions for bulimia, and may first be offered twice a week sessions.

You should initially be given group CBT sessions for binge eating disorder. If you do not find them helpful, or if you find them helpful, tell your therapist or your GP. The Person would like general counseling.

Family care. This involves working as a family with the help of a therapist through difficulties and discussing the complexities or conditions that may have triggered the feelings behind an eating disorder. It can help your family understand your issues with eating and how they can help you. People with anorexia, particularly younger people, are often offered family counseling.

Chapter 11

Safely Hypnosis Guided Weight Loss Sessions

Losing weight with hypnosis works a bit like the other change with hypnosis will. However, it's essential to know the step-by-step process so that you accurately recognize what to expect during your weight loss journey with the support of hypnosis. Generally, there are about seven steps that are involved in weight loss using hypnosis.

- The initiative is once you plan to change
- The second step involves your sessions
- The third and fourth are your changed mindset and behaviors
- The fifth step involves your regressions
- The sixth is your management routines
- The seventh is your lasting change.

To give you a far better idea of what each of those parts of your journey seems like, allow us to explore them in greater detail below.

In your initiative toward achieving weight loss with hypnosis, you've got to make a decision that you desire change, which you're willing to undertake hypnosis to vary your approach to weight loss. At now, you recognize you would like to reduce, and you've got been shown the likelihood of losing weight through hypnosis. You'll end up feeling curious, hospitable, trying something new, and a touch bit skeptical about whether this is often actually getting to work for you. You'll even be feeling frustrated, overwhelmed, or maybe defeated by the shortage of success you've got seen using other weight loss methods, which can be what leads you to hunt out hypnosis within the first place.

At this stage, the simplest thing you'll do is practice keeping an open and curious mind, as often this is how you'll set yourself up for fulfillment when it involves your actual hypnosis sessions.

Your sessions account for stage two of the method. Technically, you're getting to move from stage two through to step five several times over before you officially enter stage six. Your sessions are the stage where you engage in hypnosis, nothing more, and zip less. During your sessions, you would like to take care of your open mind and stay focused on how hypnosis can assist you. If you're struggling to remain open-minded or are still skeptical about how this might work, you'll consider switching from absolute confidence that it'll help to possess a curiosity about how it'd help instead.

Following your sessions, you're first getting to experience a changed mindset. Often this is where you begin to feel much more confident in your ability to reduce and in your ability to stay the load off. At first, your mindset should be shadowed by doubt, but as you still use hypnosis and see your results, you'll realize that you simply can create success with hypnosis. As these pieces of evidence started to point out up in your own life, you'll find your hypnosis sessions becoming even more powerful and even more successful.

In addition to a changed mindset, you're getting to start to ascertain modified behaviors. They'll be smaller initially, but you'll find that they increase over time until they reach the purpose where your expressions reflect precisely the lifestyle you've got been getting to have. The simplest part about these changed behaviors is that

they're going not to feel forced, nor will they desire you've got had to encourage yourself to urge here: your changed mindset will make these changed behaviors incredibly easy for you to settle on. As you continue performing on your hypnosis and experiencing your changed mind, you'll find that your behavioral changes grow more significant and more effortless every single time.

Following your hypnosis and your experiences with changed mindset and behaviors, you're likely getting to experience regression periods. Regression periods are characterized by periods where you start to interact in your old mindset and behavior once more. This fact happens because you've got experienced this old mindset and behavioral patterns numerous times over that they still have deep roots in your subconscious.

The more you uproot them and reinforce your new behaviors with consistent hypnosis sessions, the more success you'll have in eliminating these old behaviors and replacing them entirely with new ones. Anytime you experience the start of a regression period, you ought to put aside a while to interact during a hypnosis session to assist you in shifting your mindset back to the state that you want and wish it to be in.

Your management routines account for the sixth step, and that they inherit place after you've got adequately experienced a big and lasting change from your hypnosis practices. At now, you're not getting to got to schedule as frequent hypnosis sessions because you're experiencing such significant changes in your mindset. However, you'll still want to try to hypnosis sessions regularly to make sure that your mindset remains changed, which you are doing not revert into old patterns. Sometimes, it can take up to 3-6 months or longer with these consistent management routine hypnosis sessions to take care of your changes and stop you from experiencing a big regression in your mindset and behavior.

The final step in your hypnosis journey goes to be the step where you encounter lasting changes. At now , you're unlikely to wish to schedule hypnosis sessions any more. You ought to not got to believe hypnosis in the least to vary your mindset because you've got experienced such significant changes already, and you do not end up regressing into old behaviors. Thereupon being said, you'll find that from time to time, you would like to possess a hypnosis session to take care of your changes, particularly when an unexpected trigger may arise, which will cause you to require to regress your behaviors. These sudden changes can happen for years following your successful changes, so staying on top of them and counting on your excellent coping method of hypnosis is vital because it will prevent you from experiencing a significant regression in life.

Encourage Healthy Eating Using Hypnosis

As you undergo using hypnosis to support you with weight loss, there are a couple of ways in which you're getting to do so. One of the methods is to specialize in weight loss itself. Differently, however, is to specialize in topics surrounding weight loss. For instance, you'll use hypnosis to assist you to encourage yourself to eat healthy while also helping discourage yourself from unhealthy eating. Practical hypnosis sessions can assist you in bust cravings for foods that are getting to sabotage your success while also helping you are feeling more drawn to creating choices that are getting to assist you effectively reduce.

Many people will use hypnosis to vary their cravings, improve their metabolism, and even help themselves acquire a taste for eating healthier foods. You'll also use this to assist and encourage you to develop the motivation and energy to truly prepare healthier meals and eat them so that you're more likely to possess these healthier options available for you. If cultivating the motivation for cooking and eating healthy eating has been problematic for you, this sort of hypnosis focus is often incredibly helpful.

Using Hypnosis to Encourage Healthy Lifestyle

In addition to helping you encourage yourself to eat healthier while discouraging yourself from eating unhealthy foods, you'll also use hypnosis to assist and encourage you to form healthy lifestyle changes. This way will support you with everything from exercising more frequently to learning more active hobbies that support your wellbeing generally.

You may also use this to assist you in eliminating hobbies or experiences from your life, which will encourage unhealthy dietary habits in the first place. For instance, if you tend to scoff once you are stressed, you would possibly use hypnosis to assist you in navigating stress more effectively so that you're less likely to scoff once you are feeling stressed. If you tend to eat once you are feeling emotional or bored, you'll use hypnosis to assist you in modifying those behaviors, too.

Hypnosis is often wont to change virtually any area of your life that motivates you to eat unhealthily or otherwise neglect self-care to the purpose where you're sabotaging yourself from healthy weight loss. It truly is an incredibly versatile practice that you simply can believe, which will assist you with weight loss, also as assist you with creating a healthier lifestyle generally. With hypnosis, there are countless ways in which you'll improve the standard of your life, making it an incredibly useful practice for you to believe. You'll use hypnosis to support yourself with weight loss, also as improving your wellbeing overall.

The Right State of Mind

Find a quiet place to take a seat or lie for complete relaxation, then breathe and concentrate. Notice that the air tides in through your nostrils and the way your belly buzzes to the utmost and gently falls back to your spine as you exhale. Allow gravity to carry you securely in situ. Breathe as naturally as you'll. Don't force your breathing and notice if your breath is quick or slow and steady.

As you inhale, accept gratitude and let warmth fill your lungs. Consider the items you're grateful for. Consider something that creates you are feeling happy and peaceful. Tell yourself, "I am thankful to be alive. I'm secure and safe. I'm confident and pure." concentrate on your heart now. As you say these words to yourself, feel them deep within you. Give these statements positive energy and feed them amorously. "I love myself; I can do anything I put my mind to. I trust that my brain, body, and soul are capable of providing me with what I desire most in life."

Breathe in now and fill your mind and soul amorously and heat. Imagine as you inhale that there's a radiant light that fills your lungs before rapidly escaping your body. This light gives your patience, it gives you strength, and it provides you with the ambition and motivation to tackle the barriers that substitute your way. Exhale naturally and see as your body becomes heavier. With every breath that flows out, abandoning of negative thoughts; push those thoughts aside. You're ok, and you'll do that.

You're loved. You're special. Exhale and release all of the strain that holds you back now. What people believe and what you think are two various things. Say this far, "I believe myself."

Count your breaths now. As you inhale, breathe together with your belly and count. One, two, three, four, and five. Once you are abandoning this breath, confirm it's steady and slow. Exhale, two, three, four, five. You're accepting this positive light to vibrate through your entire being. You're letting go of all the negativity that holds you back. Inhale one, two, three, four. Exhale one, two, three, four. And inhale for one, "I am happy," two, "I am strong," three, "I am kind," four, "I am brave," five, "I am driven to succeed." exhale now. You're counting your breath from one to 5 slow and steady. Positivity embraces you now; you are feeling light and in complete control. Nothing can disturb you; nothing can bring you down; you're perfect the way you're. Repeat this step until you're able to watch your thoughts flow in and out.

Bring focus to your inner thoughts now. What pops into your mind? If you've got any negative thoughts, allow them to be there as long as they need to be without judging them. Watch them, then let them go. With every in-breath, notice your thoughts enter without judgment. These thoughts are neither positive nor negative. Once you exhale, just abandoning all hostility and anger you would possibly be holding. Let it escape into the universe and inhale, one, two, three, four, five; you're accepting all honesty and trust within yourself that you simply can make it through anything.

"I am resilient. I'm beautiful. I'm a pacesetter ."

If you notice any negative thoughts, just see them and replace them with positive, self-loving thoughts.

Breaking Barriers

Make sure that you simply are during a place where you're completely comfortable and cannot be disturbed for a minimum of thirty minutes. Have the space you're inset to a comforting temperature and confirm that the lights are low. Adjust your body so that your shoulders are relaxed, your arms are lying on either side of you, and your palms face the ceiling. You would like to become as comfortable and relaxed as you'll so that your focus isn't on your body but the meditation. Gently close your eyes and take a deep breath inward until you do not inhale. Exhale slowly and steadily so that all of the air escapes your lungs. Repeat these two more times.

Notice how your mind and body are relaxing into this guided exercise now. Breathe naturally now and convey your attention to your breath. Notice because the air fills your lungs and escapes as quickly because it entered. Breathing are some things we do a day that we frequently deem granted. It's one of the various gifts that life gives us. Just be mindful of this moment you're in immediately. Don't be concerned if your mind wanders; that's natural. There are no wrong thanks to doing that. Put trust in yourself that directly, you're not performing; you do not need to be perfect.

Bring your attention to your body and your weight now. Visualize in your mind what you appear as if and check out not to judge yourself too harshly. You're who you're, regardless of what you look as if or how you are feeling that. Erase the strain and negativity from your mind; just be present with yourself immediately.

Say to yourself

"I am beautiful. I'm strong. I can do that. I will be able to reduce, and that I won't let anyone or anything substitute my way. The sole opinion I will be able to accept is what I feel and feel about myself. At this moment and in my future moments, I think that I'm beautiful just the way that I'm ."

Let your breath suck these thoughts altogether and have your mind believe everything you tell yourself as if it had been your last wish on Earth.

As you visualize your weight immediately, I might, such as you to imagine that you are at the start of a race. There are people a bit like you're competing for fulfillment.

Say to yourself

"I got this. I will be able not to hand over. I will be able to succeed, and that I will make it to the finishing line. I will be able to conquer my fears and overcome every obstacle that stands in my way."

In the background, you hear a teacher shout, "Ready, get set..." Bring your awareness to your breath again. Inhale deeply, and as you inhale, get yourself fully committed and prepared to require your initiative toward losing weight. "Go!" exhale and visualize your feet, taking that first, second, and third breakthrough. Feel the pressure of your body depress on your legs and carry you forward. You realize this is often hard, but you do not hand over. You still jog ahead. Repeat this – "I know I can, I do know I can, I do know I can. I won't hand over; I can do that ."

You are now arising to a bicycle, and as you get thereon, you are feeling the bike hold your weight. You'll not fall. Put your feet on the pedals and begin cycling. As you cycle, you continue faster and faster. Your heart is racing from the much-needed exercise. You are feeling good. Your lungs start to harm, but you push yourself as you notice the wind flying through your hair. Notice the droplets of sweat cool your skin. You bought this, and you're coming to a curve within the course now. Turn your bike and follow the trail to the finishing line. As you reminisce, you'll see people a bit like yourself competing to end, and there are a couple of behind you and a couple of before you. While exercising, take a gentle breath in and push it out forcefully. You ought to hear a pushing sound coming from your pursed lips. Inhale and say, "I got this, I won't hand over. I will be able to succeed." you're coming to the finishing line now, but the course isn't over yet. As you cross the finishing line, you get off your bike in third place. Thanks for going!

Bring your attention now to your breath. You're breathing heavily, your heart is racing, your chest hurts, but it is a euphoric feeling. You are feeling free; you broke out of the cycle and crossed the finishing line. As you're taking a glance down your body, you notice your body has become thinner. There's a scale ahead of you on the sidelines; you've lost ten pounds. the sensation you're experiencing at this very moment is breathtaking, so you would like to undertake it again. Trust that your body knows you and what to try to. Trust in yourself that you simply will get through this.

You prepare again and wait to listen to the coach. Take a deep breath specific a count of 5 . once I count, you'll start your course. Five, four, three, two, one, and go!

Let loose your breath and feel your legs carry your ten pounds-lighter body. This point is a little more comfortable than the initial round. Your breath quickens, and your heart accelerates. You'll do that.

Say to yourself

"I will complete this course. I'm strong enough to overcome any barrier that stands in my way. This way is often hard, but nothing easy is worth doing. I got this."

In front of your now's a blow-up house with a good opening. You crawl through this opening and are covered by colorful plastic balls. They're flying at you from all angles, and it becomes hard to ascertain. Soon, you're swimming through these balls moving forward. You push these balls aside, and as you search, you see another opening. "I got this."

You tell yourself

"I will make it through, and zip can stop me now." As you reach the opening, you crawl through and are entirely on your stomach. You're during a narrow hole that you simply must army-crawl through to succeed in the top. Absorb a deep breath now. Nothing scares you. Nothing can get to you. Imagine this hole the way everyone else bullied you or picked on you. You would possibly have felt small, or enclosed, singled out, or trapped.

You have complete control, and you'll do that. You're coming closer to the sunshine at the top now. Nothing can stop you. As you reach the top of the tunnel, you leap out and begin doing jumping jacks and yell to the universe, "I did it!" You beat your fears, and you conquered the darkness, but your journey isn't over yet.

On the proper side of you, there is water on the table with a scale right next to it. You down the water and tread on the size. You notice your weight dropped another ten pounds. because the euphoric energy escapes you, you are feeling happy and delighted.

As you look before you, you see another course twenty feet away and, therefore, the finishing line at the top. Take a breakthrough now. Walk or jog at your own pace. You bought this. You've got faced harder challenges before, so you're getting to get through this one. Twenty steps later and you reach a potato sack, and five tires on the bottom laid call at a line. You jump into the potato sack, and while holding it up, you jump into the first tire hole. Take a deep breath in, and now the second tire hole. Exhale, jump into the third tire, now the fourth, and take some time. Inhale and jump into the ultimate tire.

As you leap out to end, exhale slowly. You'll feel your heart aching from the exercise. Pat yourself on the back; you're almost there. On the left side of the track, you notice weight balls that attach to your ankles and two five-pound dumbbells. You connect the ankle weights, devour the dumbbells in each hand, and appearance forward.

The finishing line is ten steps away. Take a deep breath in. "I'm almost there, I won't give up." exhale and take your initiative. The load around your ankles was an equivalent amount of weight you carried at the start of the race. You notice what proportion of a difference this is often and never want to desire this again. Take another breakthrough and feel the sweat drip down the rear of your neck. Feel the exhaustion.

Now visualize your ideal weight. Let that be your motivation to continue. With every step, you become more and more tired.

Your body becomes more and more exhausted, but you do not hand over, you retain moving forward; the finishing line just steps away now. Take a deep breath in, and there's no way you're abandoning now. You're so on the brink of your ideal weight. You've got almost accomplished your goal. You hear the people on either side of you cheer you on. Yes! You crossed the finishing line and felt that it had been all worthwhile as you step onto that scale beside you. And right before your very eyes are the numbers you've got wanted to ascertain for therefore long.

You did it! Congratulations! You're now at your ideal weight. Visualize what this seems like and absorb the thrill. Visualize what feeling you'd experience after completing your goal. Stay relaxed at this moment for as long as you'd like.

When you are ready, come to this moment. Bring your awareness to your breath. Move each finger and wiggle your toes. Feel good as you remember your visualization. You completed your goal, and you didn't hand over . that is what you'll prefer to neutralize your waking life a day. Everyone has obstacles, but you've got the willpower and now the talents to beat everyone that gets in your way. You'll open your eyes now.

Perfect Weight

"Of perfect mind and ideal weight." The terms could seem sort of fantasy to you; the sound mind and, therefore, the ideal weight. They're the realistic conditions it's possible to use as you pursue weight reduction. "Realistic?" you ask. "How can anything be 'ideal,' including my burden and my ideas about my weight?" Well, recall what we said about the facility of believing and belief.

Can it serve your curiosity to desire or hope for love or money but perfection on your own? Indulge us for a few times as we clarify why you can think your mind and burden as "perfect."

Perfect weight is the weight that's ideal for you. It is the weight that's achievable and according to everything you would like and what you're able to give yourself and accept on your own. More to the purpose, your ideal weight provides you the healthy body, the body which matches effortlessly, and also the one where you're feeling great about yourself and joyful. And what're ideal thoughts? You currently have a complete thought process, and it's flawless. But there are often a couple of ideas in those typical thoughts of yours that are providing you undesirable outcomes. There is usually something you hold in your mind, possibly habits or routines, which give you adverse outcomes. However, you'll use your ideal thoughts to align your ideas to supply you precisely what you desire. You'll use your thoughts to accomplish the bodyweight you want.

In the Twinkling of an Eye Fixed

Your current body is the outcome of your ideas and beliefs. You've acted out these ideas and feelings by the way you reside, which generated your current weight. You haven't made any errors, no matter what you'll be thinking of yourself; instead, you've just experienced undesirable outcomes. These unwanted effects are an instantaneous effect of misaligned ideas and beliefs about yourself, which are your very patterns of behavior or way of life. The Self- Hypnosis Diet is all about using your ideal thoughts to align your ideas to supply you with the results you desire. You can actually use your mind to accomplish the bodyweight you want.

Now, watch the learnings have occurred in your life, which has gotten you to where you're now together with your weight. Are you able to awaken one afternoon, and there, you're using all the extra pounds? Or was it a slow accumulation with time? Or perhaps you've understood nothing else from early youth. Regardless of the situation, many factors made your body what it's today, such as:

- Food choices
- Eating customs
- The self-critic in you
- Economic history
- Emotional background

- Influence of household
- Impact of friends
- Cultural heritage

All these and several other variables were learned in your life and eventually became your beliefs, which subsequently became patterns of activity that generated your weight. We'll be more specific and notice which those aspects appear right for you in your previous years. In other words, consider what you probably did understand in your youth about eating and food.

- What sorts of grocery did your household buy?
- What meals did your parents cook, and were they typically ready?
- Do you consume food, only reception, or does one often grab fast food?
- Have you been served fresh, healthy, home-cooked foods, or did you eat mainly processed and highly processed foods, fried foods, and "junk" foods?
- What did you understand about eating mindfully?
- Have you been taught that healthful food options led to healthy bodies?
- Did anyone teach you ways you'll understand what's healthy food and what isn't?

- Were your food selections supported, which tasted or seemed great or priced less?

Examine your own socioeconomic or sociocultural roots, and see whether or not they had an impact on the way and what you learned to consume. Over thirty-five decades back, sociological research acknowledged weight issues from the working and class consistent with their intake patterns of what has been referred to as "poverty- grade foods," like hot dogs, canned meats, and processed luncheon meats.

Cultural groups even have been analyzed to know their dietary patterns and meals, like cooking with lard or ingesting a diet of high fat and fried foods, which will cause higher body fat gain. These influences can readily be accepted because they're "normal" within the group or course. Then let's take a glance at the adolescent years. During adolescence, were there any changes in your weight? As a boy, were you invited to pile more food on your plate? "Look at him, eat more! Certainly, he's getting to become an outsized guy!" (There's a telling metaphor) Or are you currently admonished to eat? When you are a budding girl, did a sensible girl take you under her wing and ask you that the marvel of menses and, therefore, the wonderment of body modifications, as an example, organic growth in body fat with the expansion of breasts and broader shoulders?

Were you conscious during puberty, wherein, unless your body improved body fat by 22 percent, it wouldn't correctly grow and make menses? Or was that "hushed up" within a clumsy improvement? It had been likely during adolescence which you heard there is a stigma regarding obese men and ladies. Spend a few minutes writing down the aspects that appear to be accurate for you in your previous years. Ponder the encounters and influences which formed your body.

In high school, the athletes at school sports have always been a wholesome weight, so are also the cheerleaders and homecoming queens. What could ancient beliefs about your popularity and self- image have formed out of the societal interactions in high school?

What did you understand about physical activity, and what customs did you produce? Have you ever been introduced to physical activity as a part of a healthy lifestyle, through family or sports outings of walks or hikes? Or was the blaring TV a traditional fixture, enticing everybody to the sofa?

Next may be a question which most of the people haven't been conscious of during their evolution. As you're growing up, was the eye of self-care supported trendy clothes, makeup, and hairstyles, or on healthy food, routine physical activity, and spiritual and intellectual nourishment? What about today? Spend a few more minutes writing down the aspects that appear to be accurate for you within the past few decades. What influences and experiences shaped the ideas, which turned within the beliefs, which become a body?

After high school, you moved far away from home. Suddenly, you do not accept as true with your family's lifestyle.

Did you become more conscious of your options, or did you begin eating to detach steam? If you entered into an in-depth connection, what compromises or arrangements about food and physical activity, did you share input? Most relationships develop from similar pursuits, like food preferences and eating styles. Within the end, the connection comprises eating routines and tastes, which are a consequence of compromise. Have your relationships encouraged smart food choices and healthy eating? Maybe you've experienced pregnancy. Are you able to learn the thanks to getting a wholesome pregnancy and nourish a healthy infant within you? Or did you add pounds?

After parturition, did your lifestyle assist you in recovering your healthy weight or inhibit it? Within the event that you simply were active during a league or sports matches, did your livelihood or family duties take priority and eliminate these fitness activities from your regular?

Did you correct your exercise and diet? Or did the load begin to accumulate? Did an accident, injury, or illness happen that disrupted a traditional physical activity that has been supportive of a healthy weight?

It's possible to notice that how you bought and to where you're now was no accident. You heard from the parents around you and, you also collated out of the environment the way to produce food decisions. The thanks to eating, and, therefore, to taking care of yourself emotionally and physically. Whether the ideas you heard were great and healthy or not so great and not so healthy, they became your own beliefs, and eventually became you and your body because it is today. Bear in mind, you didn't do anything wrong, but you've experienced the outcomes of eating and living, which are according to your ideas and beliefs.

More than the years, what's been your answer to people and their opinions about your weight loss? bad or good? Are you able to leave and buy an incredible pair of sneakers, or did you consume more to ease the psychological distress? Maybe you even heard the latter response in your youth. Did your mom ever provide you with a plateful of food to comfort you once you felt miserable? These are learned responses, and that they are often unlearned and replaced with new answers and patterns to form your ideal weight. You ask, "Just how long does this take?" We inform you, "In the twinkle of an eye fixed ." For the minute you understand that you simply need it enough to try to anything to possess it, it's completed. You've just altered the management of highly efficient energy in you, which can be directed at deciding the way to get the result which you need: your ideal weight.

Your Perfect Mind Relearning

It isn't difficult to grasp how you bought or "heard" to weigh over your ideal weight. And it will be simple to make new decisions, to relearn new routines, and also to form new and far healthier habits. How can we learn? The simplest and most lasting learning entails repetition and practice. The most straightforward thanks to training are vital.

Pretend for a moment that you are a violinist. You're rehearsing for a grand symphony operation in NYC. Your piece includes a neighborhood of 5 pubs that's extremely hard for your fingers to perform correctly. There are two ways in which you practice. The first, which is sort of ineffective, would be to play that tough segment fast, over and over and once again, always playing the same mistakes, but trusting that your hands will play it properly

The next way is to the clinic, which can always be useful. Here, you perform the section very slowly, mindfully "teaching" your palms the thanks to maneuver, making the "muscles" ready for the acceptable moves. You are doing this steady until your palms have discovered the steps and may play the entire segment correctly and within the appropriate pace with small, if any, mindful focus.

The important thing here is that you're giving your attention to practicing correctly. By being conscious of what you're exercising, and therefore the way you're practicing it, you're studying the new patterns which are replacing the previous routines. You're practicing the action that generates your ideal weight. You, too, can create "muscle memory" by practicing mindful eating (eating slowly, chewing thoroughly, swallowing the last bite before you're taking another bite) or maybe a more cautious, slower fork-to-mouth motion. You'll even practice an entire dining design that becomes conditioned as mind-body learning or memory, which instantly becomes intuitive. Because it will become an inherent or second character, you do not get to believe doing it.

Chapter 12

Skills and Tools to Reduce Body Weight

Stimulus Control

The skill of keeping your environments stocked healthy food choices and cleared of trigger foods that make temptation.

For many years, the man spent an intrinsic part of his life chasing down food to eat. Today during a world overloaded with food choices, food is now chasing us, and it's winning.

Fat Thinking and Stimulus Control

I always ask Shift Weight Mastery Process participants to list the environments, times of day, and trigger foods they reach for. Most of their lists aren't long, but they're explanatory!

- Cheese once I return from work—with wine!
- Crackers or chips ahead of the TV.
- Eat from my boss's candy jar within the afternoon when I'm stressed.
- Eat leftover cake within the staff room.

Nine times out of ten, when a client has had an error and increased a couple of pounds, it's because of a tempting food or a specific set of meals among the environment.

Never underestimate the facility that food— especially an interesting trigger food—has on your brain and your ability to regulate it.

Trigger foods are foods that you simply can't eat just a touch of. They tend to be a food that activates your brains got to eat more and more until the bag, box, or bowl is empty.

Trigger foods also tend to be highly refined foods that contain big mouth and brain pleasers, like sugar, fat, and salt. There are exceptions to the present rule. Some people choose to spread , dried fruits, cheeses, or high-fat dairy. Any food you discover yourself circling back for or brooding about can pose a "stimulus" issue.

According to Brian Wansink, Ph.D., author of Mindless Eating, when adults are put into a state of perpetually having to decide whether or not to concede to food temptations, they get worn down and eventually concede. That's why counting on your ability to be strong and exert willpower within the presence of your favorite, fattening trigger food may be a sort of fat thinking. It just doesn't work.

Thin Thinking and Stimulus Control

Weight Masters adopt a proactive attitude with their environments instead of a defensive one. They use their minds to think on a particular level—protection. You'll cultivate thin thinking by choosing foods that are getting to be best for you in your environments and avoiding foods that challenge your weight release and maintenance.

Here are two thin thinking strategies which will make an enormous difference to your long-term weight release success:

- Stimulus-proof your environments, like your home, work, gym, car, or anywhere where you spend time and/or are susceptible to eat your trigger foods.
- Create loving boundaries together with your trigger foods.

Stimulus-Proof Your Environments

This three-part stimulus control strategy is incredibly easy in theory. Your challenge is to form it a practice.

Keep Healthy Snacks Available

You enter your front entrance after spending the last 45 minutes in traffic, and your blood glucose level is dropping as you head into the kitchen. You've got to start dinner, but as you open the fridge to tug out the salmon and salad fixings, the first things your eyes fall on are three leftover pieces of pizza. What proportion willpower does one need to assert not to stand there and erode least a couple of bites of that pizza, if not all three slices?

What if the pizza was within the back of the fridge during a covered container, and therefore the very first thing you saw was the salmon and green beans you're getting to steel oneself against dinner and a box of pea pods and cucumber slices to munch on while you cook. Because you wouldn't see the pizza, your mind isn't engaged to believe it and doesn't need to exert energy to resist it. Out of sight, out of mind, and out of mouth!

Make some extent once you shop to possess healthy snacks to succeed in for at work and reception and altogether of your environments. If you retain the healthier options upfront and simply available, your mind will stay tuned to nourishing yourself.

If a Food is Challenging You, Move It or Get and obviate It

There are a couple of ways to try to this:

- Keep challenging food out of sight. Creating a visible barrier between you and, therefore, the food sometimes is enough. I had a client who put a barrier between her and of the corn chips on the table at Mexican restaurants by placing the napkin holder and glasses to cover it. Put trigger foods in cupboards or drawers or within the back of the pantry so that they aren't in sight.

- Freeze the trigger food. This way works great for bagels, bread, cookies, and food. It removes the urge to pop some into your mouth impulsively.

- Dispose of the food. If the tactics still don't work, put the food within the garbage, and if you continue brooding about it, put the food within the trash on the road. That, my dear apprentice, is stimulus control. The rubbish disposal works well too. Remember, it's not a waste of cash if it saves you from pain and suffering. Avoiding the few hours of feeling bad about yourself is well worth the price of disposing of some trigger foods.

Stimulus-Proof Your Shopping

Millions of dollars are spent getting you to steer zombie-like down grocery aisles, putting the beautiful packages in your cart, and getting them through checkout stupidly about the later consequences to your body and your weight struggle. Don't be a pawn in their numbers game! Take back your power at the shop.

We often undermine our weight management by buying things for people at the grocery. Parents often use the excuse that "it's for the youngsters ." Two more common explanations are "what if friends come over" and "it's on sale." Shift your mind and stay focused on what you would like from the grocery. Walk by anything that you simply know are going to be calling your name later that night. Make a shopping list and stick with it!

If your Inner Rebel says, "I need to buy frozen dessert for the youngsters," but it's you who finish up eating it, expire the frozen dessert. How? Take a deep Shift Breath, connect with your thin thinking Inner Coach, and ask yourself:

- If I buy this frozen dessert, what is going to happen to it?
- Is that frozen dessert getting to be calling my name all night?
- Is that frozen dessert getting to be for the youngsters or the guests? Will I find yourself watching rock bottom of the empty carton and cursing myself for falling for the old "it's for the kids" con again?

Love yourself enough within the moment to mention "no" to the impulse. You're doing yourself an enormous favor by setting yourself free from the cravings, the food-sneaking behavior, and, therefore, the guilt after you eat it. Just walk on by. have you ever passed the frozen dessert aisle yet? Phew!

Stimulus-proofing your environments may be a potent strategy. You'll be amazed at what proportion easier weight management is when your settings are freed from the trigger foods that cause you problems.

I am not saying that you simply need to remove all the unhealthy foods or treats from your house. I'm sure many diets don't hook you. I do know that I can have bags of potato chips sitting in my cupboard for months and that I couldn't care less.

Chips don't roll in the hay on behalf me so that they don't get to leave my house. However, it's a particular issue altogether once you are talking candy and gumdrops! Those sugary candies are a trigger food on behalf of me. I do know if I even have one, I also have to eat the entire bag. So, guess what? They don't are available at my house. If they are doing, my family is under orders to not let me know. What my mind doesn't realize won't stimulate it.

Creating Loving Boundaries with your Trigger Foods

Life is long, and there'll be times once you want to enjoys an enjoyable treat, including your trigger foods. How does one set your mind up for fulfillment when having that treat? Make a rule together with your Inner Coach before time about. When and the way much of a gift you're getting to enjoy. That treat isn't an option at the other time. I call this strategy, "creating a loving boundary."

Alain Dagher, Ph.D., a neurologist at Montreal's Neurological Institute, conducted a study on expectation and brain activity concerning smoking. He measured the brain activity of smokers who were kept from smoking for four hours. One group was told that after four hours, they might smoke; the different group was told they needed to still abstain from smoking for six more hours. The smokers who expected the cigarette after four hours began to point out high levels of arousal, the closer their time to smoke came.

The other smokers, who didn't expect a cigarette, showed no arousal. When the brain knows that a gift or treat won't be forthcoming, it puts its attention elsewhere. Once you create a choice about something, and you're clear that boundary, it helps your mind say "no" comfortably.

Here's the way to roll in the hay step by step.

- Identify the trigger food. This way could be easy; it's the one you can't stop eating!

- Think of what one serving would be both in amount and calories. Confirm it allows you to remain within your Calorie allow Weight Release.

- Think of an environment during which it'd be safe to eat one serving. This environment is one that you simply haven't had a stimulus control issue in.

- Create a limit on how often you would possibly enjoy you trigger food during this setting. Creating a limit keeps you from overindulging or abusing the boundary.

For example, say your trigger food is a frozen dessert. If you didn't stop eating the frozen dessert until the carton is empty, our stimulus control strategy would be to stay frozen dessert out of your house. But what if you would like to be ready to enjoy its creamy goodness every once during a while? You'll create a replacement loving boundary with a frozen dessert.

For example, a loving boundary for frozen dessert could be "Once every week, and I can have a scoop of my favorite at the frozen dessert parlor."

You are giving yourself something you enjoy but during a moderate and measured way outside your environment. You'll even search the frozen dessert calories online and see that one scoop of rocky road is 170 calories. You'll make it work calorically for you on the day you have it, too. You've got the frozen dessert but still, remain within your Calorie allow Weight Release.

My Loving Cake Boundary

The frosting was my drug of choice once I struggled with my weight. At one wedding, I went back for five pieces of bride cake. Of course, I had to stay face. I didn't want the server to think that I used to be an out-of-control cake fiend. I told him that I used to be bringing the additional slices to others at my table. Little did he know that the others at my table were my Inner Rebel and her wild friends partying on cake deep inside me!

As I started my journey to weight mastery, I created a healthy and loving boundary around the cake that works on behalf of me still. I tell myself, "Cake and frosting on behalf of me isn't an option unless it's my birthday or the birthday of anyone in my immediate family."

This fundamental rule around the cake may be a perfect fit for me. For every family member's birthday, I will be able to make a cake and have an exquisite piece with extra icing. In my inner rule system, the cake isn't an option unless it's my birthday or my husband's and children's birthdays.

Create Your Trigger Food Loving Boundary

Exercise

Take a flash to fill in your trigger foods and make a loving boundary.

- Stimulus-proof your environments by removing the trigger foods that tempt you and having healthy choices available, once you aren't falling victim to high-calorie foods in your situation, it's much easier to remain consistently on target with weight release.

- Bringing healthy food into your environments and having them available for meals and snacks is different to make sure your situation is about up to assist you in succeeding.

- Create loving mental boundaries around your favorite trigger foods so that you'll have them in your life occasionally but in a controlled way. Knowing your trigger foods and creating a masterful relationship with them puts you responsible.

- Stimulus control is a crucial skill not just for releasing weight but also for long-term weight management.

APPRENTICE PAUSE: have you ever felt protective of somebody or something? Perhaps you've got cared for a little child or a pet? It's quite an intense feeling, right? Why is it that when it involves your self-care and weight, you don't step in to guard yourself?

Now that you simply understand the skill of stimulus control, you'll be your protector, bringing a replacement level of self-protection to your life within the way you're taking care of yourself and, therefore, the environments you reside in.

Weight Loss Hypnosis

To start this hypnosis, confirm that you simply are during a comfortable position. Don't attempt to do that once you are driving and wait to try to it publicly, like on a bus or a plane. You are doing not skills your body might react, so it's best if you're focused on doing this reception while on your couch, or perhaps as you're falling asleep. Remove all other distractions and focus only on staying comfortable. Focus only on your breathing and hear the subsequent directions as you begin to fall under a relaxed state.

For this hypnosis, you're getting to visualize what's waiting ahead of you. Let the thoughts flow through your mind as if they're your own.

Everything that we are getting to discuss during this motivation is about you, and only you. We are getting to begin with "I" statements because these are affirmations. These are the thoughts you would like to urge into your head to rewire the way that you only are thinking towards something more positive and healthier.

I am inhaling and that I can feel myself fill with life because the air enters my body. Because it comes, I count one, two, three, four, and five. Because it exists, I count six, seven, eight, nine, ten. Counting my breath helps me to manage it. When my breathing is regulated, everything else in my body is going to be also. These processes are reliable, and that I understand that my body is capable of anything.

I have begun to concentrate on the items that I'm eating to assist me in reducing. Within the past, I used to be unhealthier and that I made poor decisions for my body.

This way has led me to where I have gained weight, and now, I feel unhappy with the person who I even have become.

I have tried to reduce it within the past. I even have considered eating foods that are bad on my behalf and that I may need also considered some unhealthy dieting methods, like crash dieting or harmful pills.

I did this because I used to be taught to hate my body. I wanted to punish myself for the shape that I had found myself in after making more unhealthy choices. I made unhealthy decisions to undertake and reduce, not that specialize in my psychological state within the process.

These unhealthy choices led me to an area of negative thinking. I feel bad thoughts about my body, which only makes it harder on behalf of me to reduce.

At this moment, I'm getting to stop this negative thinking. I will be able not to be focused on hurting or punishing myself anymore.

The only thing I care about is ensuring that I'm a healthy person. I'm focused when it involves my health and, therefore, the foods that I'm putting into my body. I care about the wealthy , but I care even more about feeling better.

I am uninterested in trying a new diet after a new diet. Each new thing I discover, I buy small hope, but it fails. It doesn't fail due to the meal plan, but due to my mindset. I buy frightened of what is going to happen once I fail, so I'd not even try within the beginning.

I am not getting to allow myself to think like this anymore. I'm only getting to be focused on positive thinking and a healthy mindset to assist within the achievement of my goals.

I don't want to urge stuck within the same thinking pattern for the remainder of my life. I deserve better. I deserve entirely just hating my body. I need to be happy from the within, which will start to point out on the surface.

I am always surprised at how hard my body works because it consistently exceeds my expectations. Once I am sick, I'm wondering if I will be able ever to feel better, but my body does most of the add fighting things off. I'm ready to achieve great things with my body, and therefore the only reason I'd have fallen off my healthy lifestyle path within the past is that I did not see that initially.

Going forward, I'm getting to be focused on seeing the fantastic things that I'm capable of. I'm only curious about tracking the items that I even have done. I'm not focused on the topics that I'm still waiting to accomplish. I'm grounded within the "now," because that's the sole thing that matters to me during this weight loss journey.

I am centered with my body, and I'm determined to urge it to the right place. I'm not getting to try anything harmful to reduce. Instead, I'm getting to work with my body, not against it. I'm getting to use the tools that are the foremost helpful in ensuring that I reduce successfully, so I don't need to worry about it returning on later in life.

I am taking a positive path towards getting the items that I desire. I felt like weight loss took goodbye before. Often this is because I used to be tracking my progress multiple times each day. Within the past, if I didn't see results within a few days, then I might think that something wasn't right.

I understand now that this was just a mentality that was taught to me. My body works much faster than I'm ready to see, but I wont to only measure it by the items that were happening on the surface.

Moving forward, I'm only focused on measuring progress with how good I feel. Accepting this mentality alone makes me feel better already. once I am clearly focused on ensuring that my psychological state is that the most vital, then everything else seems such a lot easier.

The reason weight-loss felt love it took goodbye within the past was because I used to be impatient. I understand how time works now and that I realize that I can't track things as closely as I want to. Within a month, I will be able to see far more progress than what's seen during a day, and that I understand the difference now.

I am understanding of how I want to twiddle my thumbs, and the way this mentality will help me to reduce rapidly. If I buy too impatient, I will be able to attempt to rush a process that takes time, and it'll only make it feel longer within the end.

I am not getting to give my attention to fast weight loss. I am getting to ignore the size.

I will only specialize in numbers during a long-term sense, like

monthly weigh-ins.

I am getting to be the foremost concerned with how I'm feeling mentally.

If I ignore how I feel mentally, then this may only hold me back further and keep me within the place that I'm already trying so desperately to urge out of.

I am not getting to fight against my body anymore. I'm only getting to confirm that I'm using its natural processes to reduce. Once I am often patient, it'll make the load loss feel much faster.

I am getting to keep track of my weight loss reasonably, and I'm getting to drop the unrealistic expectations that I've created for myself.

I am getting to be compassionate to myself during this process. I understand that I will be able to make some mistakes.

I have the motivation and encouragement needed within myself to form sure that I don't let these mistakes become defining moments in my life.

Each time I feel as if I even have slipped far away from a goal, I will be able to remember that it's up to me to urge back on target from an area of determination and dedication.

I am getting to be forgiving of myself for my natural urges and need to follow old habits.

I am getting to be more reliable than the person who I used to be within the past, but I also remember that they're still strong themselves.

I am focused only on living a healthy lifestyle and losing weight rapidly. I understand that thanks to making this process fast is to stay to it. There are not any shortcuts or quick fixes. This way is often a process that's getting to be a lifelong journey, but that doesn’t mean I can’t still see results within a comparatively close time-frame.

I understand that being patient and sticking this diet out is what's getting to help me reduce the quickest.

I accept the very fact that I cannot rush this process and need to take it because it comes. My body knows what it's doing and that I trust that it's the facility to form up for the items that I cannot control. I’m getting to encourage my body to reduce through keto and fasting, but it'll still be up to my body what proportion weight I will be able to lose and at what pace.

I will not compare my body to others anymore. I’m only focused on myself and that I know that I even have all the facilities needed to seek out success.

As I continue during this hypnosis, I’m reminded of where I’m now and where I will be able to be going next. I’m getting to count to 10, and once I reach ten, I will be able to be out of the meditation and either drifting to sleep or back within the world where

I’m more focused and prepared to lose the load. My breathing remains regulated and can still plan the hypnosis has ended. One, two, three, four, five, six, seven, eight, nine, ten.

Weight Loss Tips and Tricks

To achieve your weight loss goals, you want to be willing to let any fear and doubt you'll have about hypnotherapy, go. It's not something that you simply can second guess, particularly not its effectivity and results-driven orientation. It's an answer used for several different reasons, even aside from weight loss. Hypnotherapy for weight loss can assist you in overcoming a negative relationship with food, one which will have formed over a period or throughout your entire life. It's something which will present you with proper results which you'll always be sure of.

Although it's not a diet or weight loss supplement, it fulfills an identical supporting role and is the inspiration on the journey of living a more mindful lifestyle. Since the tactic thereof is concentrated on replacing old negative habits with new positive ones, it helps one to beat challenges faced when trying to reduce.

Whether you would like to choose a one-on-one weight loss for hypnotherapy session or simply hear audiobooks online, both can serve you usefully.

Before you dive into the planet of hypnotherapy, you ought to know that there are tons more to it than you'll have initially thought. Very similar to Yoga and meditation, generally, it serves a greater purpose because it leads you on to a mindful path of physical, mental, and emotional wellness.

Chapter 13

Tips for a rapid Weight Loss Hypnosis

Find the proper hypnotherapist for weight loss for you. How would you set about doing this, you'll ask? Rather than going the obvious route of checking out hypnotherapists online in your area, why not invite recommendations instead? Honestly, what's better than asking a lover, loved one, or acquaintance to recommend you an honest hypnotherapist for weight loss? If nobody you recognize knows a hypnotherapist that's known for the outstanding jobs they perform, then you'll want to see together with your doctor and invite advice. They ought to be ready to recommend a professional and results- oriented hypnotherapist for weight loss. To make sure you've got the proper hypnotherapist, make certain to see with yourself whether their consultation felt as if it had been thorough. Know if the hypnotherapy program is adjusted to satisfy your needs and also if the practitioner helped answer your questions. Once they leave space between sessions, it shows you're handling an honest hypnotherapist.

Don't Pay Any Attention to Advertising

We sleep in 2020, which suggests that everything we see online is taken seriously. However, it should not be. People are oblivious and vulnerable to accept everything they read or hear, but when it involves advertising, not everything is often trusted.

Advertising should, ever often, be disregarded and not taken too seriously because it is often very misleading. It is usually better to conduct your research before you merely accept that something may be a certain way or not. Within the case of hypnotherapy, since there are

numerous negative associations associated with the practice, it is best to seek out what's it all about yourself. As you'll see from this handy set of data provided about hypnotherapy for weight loss, it's completely safe and doubtless nothing negative that you simply expected it to be.

Get Information About Training, Qualifications, And Necessary Experience

Before you choose a hypnotherapist, you want to make sure about their necessary information first. You want to know: Do they run the practices together or operate independently? Are they certified and have a license? Ensuring that they also adhere to moral standards, most preferably recommended by other medical physicians, you will be assured that you simply are handling someone who knows what they're doing.

Before Choosing One Hypnotherapist, Ask

Several First

One of the simplest ways to seek out whether a hypnotherapist is best fitted to you is to speak with a couple of them over a call first. This way may take some effort, but it'll be worthwhile within the end. You've got to think about whether or not they can relate to you, care about your wellbeing, and hear your concerns, whether or not they are personable, accommodating, and professional. If they tick all the boxes, then you're good to travel.

Don't Fall for Any Unrealistic Promises

If a hypnotist tells you that their therapy session will assist you in reducing fast, then don't even bother getting to one session. Hypnosis for weight loss may be a process that takes time. It can take anywhere between three weeks, up to 3 months, to ascertain your human body change and to reduce. Since your body and mind should first adjust, you would like to permit time for it to try to so. Hypnosis for weight loss isn't a fad; neither is it a way of losing weight overnight. It is also essential to avoid hypnotherapists who suggest they're going to cause you to reduce. Since they're going only to be talking during the session, what they're telling you isn't true whatsoever. What you'll expect from a knowledgeable and authentic hypnotherapist, however, maybe a professional individual who takes responsibility for helping you to urge where you would like to travel. This person should assist you in accessing your subconscious with ease and assist you in bringing it on board with a correct weight loss plan and possibly an exercise routine.

Is Your Hypnotherapist of Choice Multi- Skilled?

Even though hypnosis may be a terrific tool and may alter the mind's way of brooding about food, it goes hand-in-hand with nutrition. This way is often something you would like to think about, mainly whether your hypnotist features a good understanding of what it takes for you to reduce sustainably and healthily. Many of us focused on starting a weight loss journey don't necessarily know what they ought to do or what they ought to eat. When trying to find a hypnotherapist, search for one that features a self-help coaching or some sort of

psychotherapy qualification, also as a qualification/background in either nutrition or cognitive behavioral therapy.

Find Out the Time You Ought to Engage During A Program

This therapy is quite important as hypnotherapy can become quite expensive if you are going to knowledgeable for one-on-one sessions. If you favor getting to knowledgeable instead of conducting the courses at your home, you'll prefer to spread your sessions out over time to form it cheaper. Albeit you'll think that the sessions subsided effective in achieving the general effect, it works more effectively as your mind and body require time to regulate. Time is additionally required as you modify your old habits and replace them with new ones to reduce.

Questions to Ask

- Ask your hypnotherapist if they will provide you with a program to take care of your progress reception. A recording mainly helps to permit you to opened up sessions over time. Taking note of your weight loss hypnosis recording a day will keep you in restraint and assist you to stay motivated and focused.

As your hypnotherapist, if they will tailor-make your hypnotherapy weight loss program for you. If the therapist complies with it, you'll expect a weight loss hypnotherapy program that's far more effective than individualized hypnosis, offering treatments that will work better than ones that cater to everyone. Since everyone is different compared to others, this makes tons more sense. Sure, the overall program will work, but a customized one could provide you with better results.

- Ask whether your program includes an introduction session. Starting with hypnotherapy for weight loss, you do not want to only dive right into it. It is vital to require the required time, albeit it's just an hour, to determine your needs and concerns regarding your current habits, lifestyle, and goals together with your hypnotherapist. Ensuring that they care about your wellbeing and results rather than just taking you thru the session is equally important. Taking the time to speak to your therapist and going to know them better will assist you to feel more comfortable and form a foundation of trust before starting together with your hypnotherapy sessions.

Establish the prices involved before starting together with your sessions.

Ensuring you recognize what proportion an initial consultation and every session cost are going to be another important factor you've got to think about before choosing a hypnotherapist. Considering the worth, a summary of the therapist program compared to other potential weight loss programs. Review supported the standard of service you'll receive, and take under consideration that you simply can spread your practice over weeks rather than getting to a couple of sessions every week.

Lastly, you ought to view hypnotherapy as an investment in yourself and wellbeing, instead of an unnecessary expense. The context for this thought will realize once you engage in or complete your program.

Tips for Managing Stress to Avoid Emotional Eating

No matter what your binge eating cycles are like, stress is nearly bound to encourage you to interact in emotional eating. When it involves stress and its ability to influence your dietary behaviors, there are generally two ways in which it can happen.

The first is that you simply end up feeling stressed, and you binge eat as how to make some sort of comfort in your life so that you're not feeling quite as stressed anymore. The opposite way includes you feeling so stressed that you simply think that you cannot eat, then binge eating when your body cannot take the stress-induced fasting anymore. In either scenario, stress can negatively affect your diet and may also become a negative coping method that worsens your binge eating within the future, too. Furthermore, both of those behavioral patterns around stress and eating can cause weight gain, which suggests that they're not productive to your goals of weight loss.

Managing stress to avoid emotional eating largely revolves around you learning the way to deal with and manage your stress properly. The more proactive you'll be in handling your pressure, the less likely you're to hunt out behaviors like binge eating as a chance to assist you to overcome the strain that you simply are experiencing.

People who routinely experience problematic binge eating, thanks to stress or other emotions, will often address healthier practices like meditating, preventative self-care, and routine relaxation practices to

assist them in reducing stress. This way, they're less likely to interact in emotional eating within the first place.

When it involves handling bursts of upper-stress levels, meditating is often incredibly helpful in assisting you with bringing your stress levels to backtrack. This way, you're more likely to feel asleep and less susceptible to feel the necessity to affect your stress through less healthy means, like through overeating.

Preventative self-care measures that will assist you in affecting your stress are incredibly useful in avoiding stress within the first place. For instance, budgeting more effectively so that you're not so worried about money, creating a bank account, exercising daily, and spending time with loved ones are all great ways to avoid scenarios where your stress may rise unnecessarily.

The simpler you're at handling areas of your life that typically end in stress, the simpler you'll be in eliminating your stress. Or, when it can't be removed, a minimum of minimizing it so that you'll feel more asleep in your life.

Routine relaxation practices are almost like preventative self-care, except that they're more focused on the day to day practices that are meant to assist you to relax regardless of what has triggered your stress.

For example, some people click after work a day and luxuriate in a while gardening, reading a book, or just resting on the couch with their eyes closed so that they need time to decompress from the day they need had. People wish to take a candlelit bath, choose a walk, or maybe play a game on their laptop as how to destress. The thought here is that you simply find a good thanks to decompressing whenever you are feeling stressed, which you are doing it on a day to day in order that your stress doesn't begin to rise an excessive amount of within the first place.

When it involves managing your stress to avoid overeating, the simplest thing you'll do is still try new routines and rituals until you discover practices that assist you in destressing without overeating.

The exact “formula” for destressing is going to be different for everybody, so you're getting to need to take a while to seek out that information out for yourself. The higher you understand your own needs around stress and the way to relax, the more likely you're to be ready to come up with a practice that's getting to assist you in destressing in the first place.

Chapter 14

Introduction to Intermittent fasting

If your goal is to lose weight, as is the case with so many women, you will find detailed information on how intermittent fasting leads to weight loss and tips that you can employ to lose weight faster. You will also learn that the benefits of this regimen go far beyond weight loss; you also significantly reduce the risk factors of a host of lifestyle diseases, most of which have been covered here. If you're already a victim of such diseases, this book is for you too. You will be informed on how to fast, and how fasting will help you deal with your illness. You will be glad to know that many women have found relief in intermittent fasting. This information has been compiled after extensive research from various sources, as well as testimonials from participants who have experienced intermittent fasting. It gives practical guidelines that any woman can follow with satisfactory results. Practice due caution when undertaking procedures suggested in this book. The information is accurate to the best of the writer's knowledge, but the results could vary depending on individual circumstances. This is however not medical content, and should any issue arise, don't hesitate to consult a doctor. You're advised not to substitute your prescribed medication with the remedies suggested here. Ask the doctor if you can use the two concurrently, or if you have to finish with your medication first. That said, it is my sincere hope that you'll find this content of value and will pick up practical tips that you can apply in your weight loss journey. Happy reading! Please note that the contents of this book are under copyright, and the duplication of any part of it without written permission from the publisher is prohibited

Intermittent fasting refers to an eating pattern where you alternate between phases of eating and fasting. This method does not concentrate much on the foods that should be eaten or avoided, but rather when the food should be eaten. You can abstain from food partially or entirely, depending on your ability and your needs. If the fasting is partial, you can take a little amount of food mostly fruits and vegetables whose calorie content does not exceed 500. You can also sip on non-caloric drinks such as water, black coffee or black tea. Intermittent fasting gives your digestive system time to rest. Think about it, if you eat every 4 to 5 hours, your digestive tract to be always burdened. Once you give it a break, it ends up metabolizing faster and burning more calories. Faster metabolism coupled with reduced calorie intake results in weight loss, one of the key benefits of intermittent fasting.

Intermittent fasting is as old as mankind itself. As long as humans have existed, they have often fasted periodically for one reason or the other whether voluntarily or forced by circumstances. Reasons for fasting range from lack of food to religious and health reasons. In the present-day world, the precise benefits of fasting have been studied since the early 2000s. Intermittent fasting, in particular, showed several benefits and quickly gained a following. In 201, the media picked up the debate interviewing scores of people whose lives have been transformed by the fast. Since then, many people have turned intermittent fasting into a lifestyle and have a lot to show for it.

Types of Intermittent Fasting plans

It can be categorized into different kinds depending on the mode of fasting. How long should you fast? This part is very important since you're dealing with an eating plan that concentrates on the timelines of eating and not eating. Think of intermittent fasting as simply skipping meals; which is what it is in the simplest of terms. Here we look at the different arrangements of skipping meals. Your style of fasting would be determined by your individual needs. Intermittent fasting should not strain you unnecessarily; remember this is more of a lifestyle change than a diet.

Here at the regiment that you can choose from:

1. Skipping Meals

If you're just starting out, this is a good point to begin. Skip a meal or two every once in a while. Think of it; even without planning we all get to skip a meal every now and then. Now do this consciously, looking at each missed meal as an opportunity to ease into fasting mode. If you are traveling, resist the urge to stop for a meal. Work through lunch break. Skip breakfast when running late. If there's hardly anything to cook in the house, don't order in. If you're not hungry, don't force down a meal for the sake of it. Just keep busy and let mealtime slide by. What better way to fast without feeling deprived? When you finally do eat, go for a healthy meal to avoid reversing the benefits of fasting.

2. 12 Hour Fast

Staying without food for 12 hours sounds like a tall order until you include sleep into the schedule. When you are asleep, you're already fasting, right? If you sleep for 8 hours, say from 10 pm to 6 am, you only have 4 hours left. You can then skip breakfast and have brunch at 10 am. Alternatively, you can have an early dinner and start fasting by 6 pm. By the time you get up at 6 am, your fasting window will be over. It is actually quite simple, and friendly for beginners 3. 16 Hour Fast This is one of the most common fasting regimens, also called the 16:8 method referring to the fasting timelines. It is also referred to as the Leangains diet. If you have successfully attempted the 12-hour fast, you can now proceed to this 16 hour one. Some experts suggest that the number of hours can be modified to 14 or 15 hours. The 16-hour rule here was formulated with men in mind, and it is universally agreed that women can make the first 1 or 2 hours shorter. However, should you be able to cover the 16 hours without feeling excessively hungry or weak, go right ahead. How can you achieve 16 hours of fasting? Eat your dinner by 9 pm, skip breakfast the following morning and have your lunch at 1 pm. You can break the fast an hour or two earlier if you so choose. 16 hours sound like such a long time without food, but you're essentially skipping just one meal. When you think of it like that, it actually sounds achievable.

4. Alternating Days

This plan involves fasting every other day. You eat one day, fast the next, eat the following one and so on. Since most people will not manage an entire 24 hours without eating, some versions of this plan allow the 9 consumption of up to 500 calories in the fasting period. Given that women are supposed to take about 2000 calories per day, this means reducing your intake to only 1/4 of the ordinary. Fasting for 24 hours with no mean feat. Alternate day fasting is only recommended for those who have been fasting for some time and have gotten accustomed to it. Beginners will find it a bit extreme. If you have a health condition or are on medication, consult your doctor before embarking on this plan. Alternate day fasting also scores low in terms of sustainability. Perhaps it is possible that your lifestyle will not allow you to keep fasting for entire days, especially if your job demands a substantial amount of physical or emotional energy. You should be in a position to plan your days according to your fasting schedule, as it is important for your weight loss goals.

5. 2 Day Fast (Eat Stop Eat Method)

You can fast 2 days a week, separating them with a couple of days eating window. This means the fasting days are not executive, of course, you won't be expected to go for 48 hours without food. Just pick any two days that suit you. It could be Monday and Thursday, Wednesday and Friday, Thursday and Saturday and so on. Should you be hard pressed during the fasting days, you can consume a maximum of 500 calories to keep you going. A for the eating days, maintain a normal healthy diet. There are various means of achieving a 24 hour fast. Think of it as a breakfast to breakfast, lunch to lunch or dinner to dinner fast provided you take those meals at a similar time. If you had your dinner at 8 p.m., then break the fast at 8 pm the following day. The same applies for the other meals. You can have non-caloric beverages in the fast period or small low- calorie meals. This plan is also known as the 5:2 referring to the weekly number of eating and fasting days.

6. The Warrior Meal Plan

Here the eating window is restricted to a period of 4 hours only. This one is definitely not for beginners; you need some practice first before you can go for 20 hours without food. The warrior diet allows you to eat some little food during the day, normally just fruits and raw vegetables, then eat a large meal at night. Some people swear by this method, reasoning that one large meal is enough to fuel the body for 20 hours. Indeed, with a meal containing plenty of proteins, vegetables, and healthy fats, it is possible to cover the 20-hour fast window without much strain.11 There are opponents though, who argue that a large meal at dinner time makes it hard to sleep. Both opinions are valid. Feel free to try various fasting techniques until you find the one best suited for your needs.

Conclusion

This book may be a blend of all the effective techniques to assist people that are affected by excessive weight gain. It presents a special dimension of how the key to weight loss lies in your brain. It covers the techniques of self-hypnosis, Cognitive behavioral therapy (CBT), Sleep Learning, and Meditation. All of those techniques request active involvement of the brain and alter within the wiring pattern of the mind. In this way, it is possible to boost a satisfactory level of the brain to prevent the urges of overeating. The book contains an in-depth account of all the activities, processes, and requirements to form of these techniques healthily compute for you.

This book serves multiple purposes. It not only guides about weight loss techniques but also the basis causes of the opposite emotional problems that promote overeating. This book is a complete guide to a fatless, healthy, happy, and satisfactory lifestyle.

CPSIA information can be obtained
at www.ICGtesting.com
Printed in the USA
BVHW082313030521
606340BV00007B/1799

9 781802 340624